*The*
# Superpowers!
*of*
*Therapeutic*
# Fasting

*Ancient Advice and Medical Miracles*

Frank Marrero, *Enelysios*

*with* Upton Sinclair's *The Fasting Cure*

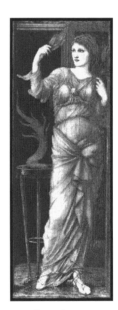

Tripod Press

This book, like my whole life,
is dedicated to Avatar Adi Da, Samraj,
whom I am graced to call Beloved.

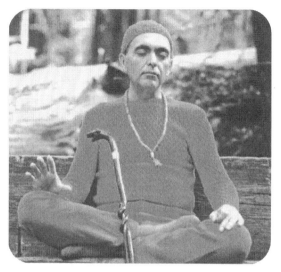

*Shown here in 1986 during his 150 day fast.*

# Table of Contents

## Preface: The End of Authority

The core of this book is found in the second chapter, "Words of the Day: Pluripotency / Autophagy". The latest medical research about fasting delivers an acuity of understanding and awe-filled scientific revelation like never before. No longer do we need to wonder about the bio-chemical and systemic effects associated with all modalities of fasting. No longer do we need to believe authorities who promote their provincial beliefs, limited interpretations, or personal agenda with regards to fasting: it's science now, *combined with our own informed and direct experience.* We can simply listen to antecdotal advice and trail-blazers and winnow what makes sense to us. The end of authority begins with grounded understanding and our own responsibility.

Fortunately, the research is clear—while ironically bordering on miraculous. Unfortunately, the most recent science is not easy to take in. This fact inspired me to attempt an explanation for the lastest findings. Everything else in this book is just a kind of "good company" surrounding and supporting the **Words of the Day**.

This is not a "how to" book, even as there are bits of wisdom one may gather. If you are new to fasting (check with your doctor of course), you can take in *The Idiot's Guide to Fasting* along with Michael Mosley's "5-2" books (see *The FastDiet - Revised & Updated: Lose Weight, Stay Healthy, and Live*

*Longer with the Simple Secret of Intermittent Fasting*), and wander around the myriad of *www.fasting.com* or the simpler *www.allaboutfasting.com* for starters.

You will see, as the science clearly shows, that a myriad of fasts all have great benefit. With every kind and level of fasting, the corresponding depth of benefits can now be understood. The good news is that the most modest and easiest approaches have most of the benefits.

Pick the kind of approach you think best, or experiment. They're all great, for with each style you learn the dance of chosen hunger. When you can do that two-step on the dancefloor, superpowers begin.

This is a news flash. Before dismissing fasting as something you can't do, check out the latest science and how easy it can be.

If you want it quick and effortless, invest 57 minutes and take in the BBC Documentary, "Eat, Fast, and Live Longer," available for free outside the Queen's domain.

https://www.youtube.com/watch?v=Ihhj_VSKiTs

*This documentary includes interviews with this book's main living heroes, Dr. Victor D. Longo (Edna M. Jones Professor of Gerontology and the Biological Sciences at the USC Davis School of Gerontology and director of the USC Longevity Institute) and Mark P. Mattson (Director of the National Institute on Aging Intramural Research Program, National Institutes of Health, Department of Neuroscience, Johns Hopkins University School of Medicine).*

Having taken in the science, you can more easily navigate the challenges that superpowers require.

But like we did upon entering the ancient healing center at Epidavros, founded by Asklepios with his Caduceus, let us first listen to the trailblazers before us and take in the accounts from lasting voices, ancient and modern, about the powers of healing and fasting.

# A World of Praise for Fasting

Man lives on one quarter of what he eats; on the other three quarters lives his doctor.
— Pyramid Inscription (5800 years old!)

He who buries his head deep into a nose-bag full of food cannot hope to see the invisible world.
— Al Ghazzali

There's a hidden sweetness in the stomach's emptiness.
We are lutes, no more, no less.
If the sound box is stuffed full of anything, no music.
If the brain and the belly are burning clean with fasting,
every moment a new song comes out of the fire.
The fog clears, and a new energy makes you run up the steps
in front of you.
Fasting is the first principle of medicine. Fast and see the
strength of the spirit reveal itself.
Fasting blinds the body
in order to open the eyes of your soul.
Fasting is an amazing thing.
It gives people heart and soul.
If you want to ascend like the Prophet
to the sky of immortality,
know this very well:
Fasting is your Arabian stallion.
— Rumi (trans. Nevit O. Ergin)

He that never eats too much will never be lazy.
Dine with little, sup with less, do better still, sleep supperless.
To lengthen thy life, lessen thy meals.
Nine in ten deaths are suicides.
The best of all medicines are rest and fasting.
— Benjamin Franklin


Men do not die, they kill themselves.
— Seneca


Very few people know what real health is, because most are occupied with killing themselves slowly.
— Albert Szent-Gyorgyi, Ph.D Biochemistry; Nobel Prize in physiology and medical science


To refuse food and drink is more than a pleasure; it is the joy of the soul!
— Leo Tolstoy


One can have no smaller or greater mastery than mastery of oneself.
— Leonardo da Vinci, fasting practitioner


Start the practice of self-control with some penance; begin with fasting.
— Mahavira (Founder of Jainism)

Fasting and prayer are religious exercises; the enjoining them, an act of discipline.
— Thomas Jefferson

A little starvation can really do more for the average sick man than can the best medicines and the best doctors. I do not mean a restricted diet; I mean total abstinence from food. I speak from experience; starvation has been my cold and fever doctor for 15 years, and has accomplished a cure in all instances… A little starvation can really do more for the average sick man than can the best medicines and best doctors.
— Mark Twain

Fasting is a natural method of healing. When animals or savages are sick, they fast.
— Paramahansa Yogananda

Take away food from a sick man's stomach and you have begun, not to starve the sick man, but the disease.
— E. H. Dewey, M.D

So he was there with the Lord forty days and forty nights; he did not eat, and he wrote on the tablets the words of the covenant, the Ten Commandments.
— Exodus 34:28

I fast for greater physical and mental efficiency.
— Plato

Seest thou what fasting does: it heals illnesses, drives out demons, removes wicked thoughts, makes the heart pure. If someone has even been seized by an impure spirit, let her or him know that this kind, according to the word of the Lord, 'goeth not out but by prayer and fasting.'
    — Matthew 17:21

The soul breath of the fasting man's mouth is more fragrant before God and better pleasing to Him than a redolent monk... Prayer takes us half-way towards God, fasting takes us to the gates of Heaven.
    — Mohammed

Fasting possesses great power. If practiced with the right intention, it makes one a friend of God. The demons are aware of that.
    — Quintus Tertullian

O ye who believe, fasting is prescribed for you … as it was prescribed for those before you, so that you may safeguard yourselves against every kind of ill and become righteous.
    — Quran

Fasting men and fasting women, God has prepared forgiveness and a splendid wage.
    — Quran-AlAhzab

Fasting cures diseases, dries up bodily humors, puts demons to flight, gets rid of impure thoughts, makes the mind clearer and the heart purer, the body sanctified, and raises man to the throne of God.

— Athenaeus of Naucratis

The philosophy of fasting calls upon us to know ourselves, to master ourselves, and to discipline ourselves the better to free ourselves. To fast is to identify our dependencies, and free ourselves from them.

— Tariq Ramadan

In a fast we can observe the body gleefully going about getting rid of toxins and wastes accumulated for years with the greatest capability and intelligence, all on its own.

— William Esser MD

Juice fasting is, without any doubt, the most effective biological method of treatment. It is the 'operation without surgery.' It is a cure involving exudation, re-attunement, redirection, loosening up and purified relaxation. While fasting, the patient improves her or his physical health and gains much, but he or she will have neglected the most important thing if the hunger for spiritual nourishment that manifests itself during fasting is not satisfied. When the body fasts, the soul is hungry.

— Otto Buchinger, Sr., M.D

I believe that fasting is the "missing link" in the Western diet...
Fasting is the single greatest natural healing therapy. It is
nature's ancient, universal 'remedy' for many problems.
— Elson Haas, M.D.

Everyone can perform magic, everyone can reach his goals, if
he is able to think, if he is able to wait, if he is able to fast.
— Hermann Hesse, Siddhartha

Through fasting, let your mind depend on its own power.
When that power manifests, the life force in the body becomes
increasingly reinforced with the eternal energy continually
flowing into the brain and spine from the cosmic energy
around the body, entering through the medulla. Becoming
detached from dependence on outer, physical sources of bodily
sustenance, the life force sees that it is being supported from
within, and wonders how this is so. The mind then says: 'The
solids on which the body used to depend are nothing more
than gross condensations of energy. You are pure energy, and
you are pure consciousness.'
— Paramahansa Yogananda

Fasting is the master key to mental and spiritual unfoldment
and evolution.
— Dr. Arnold Ehret

Fasting of the body is food for the soul.
— John Chrysostom

Whether the patient has a cardiac condition, hypertension, autoimmune disease, fibroids, or asthma, he or she must be informed that fasting and natural, plant-based diets are a viable alternative to conventional therapy, and an effective one... The body's wondrous ability to autolyze (or self-digest) and destroy needless tissue such as fat, tumors, blood vessel plaque, and other nonessential and diseased tissues, while conserving essential tissues, gives the fast the ability to restore physiologic youth to the system. By removing or lessening the burden of diseased tissue, including the fatty tissue narrowing the blood vessels, fasting increases the blood flow and subsequent oxygenation and nutrient delivery to vital organs throughout the body.
— Joel Fuhrman, M.D.

Abstinence and fasting cure many a complaint.
— Danish Proverb

He who eats until he is sick must fast until he is well.
— English Proverb

Fasting is the support of our soul: it gives us wings to ascend on high, and to enjoy the highest contemplation! God, like an indulgent father, offers us a cure by fasting.
— Saint John Chrysostom

I do, by this my proclamation, designate and set apart Thursday, the 30th day of April, 1863, as a day of national humiliation, fasting and prayer. And I do hereby request all the People to abstain, on that day, from their ordinary secular pursuits, and to unite, at their several places of public worship and their respective homes, in keeping the day holy to the Lord, and devoted to the humble discharge of the religious duties proper to that solemn occasion.

All this being done, in sincerity and truth, let us then rest humbly in the hope authorized by the Divine teachings, that the united cry of the Nation will be heard on high, and answered with blessings, no less than the pardon of our national sins, and the restoration of our now divided and suffering Country, to its former happy condition of unity and peace.

In witness whereof, I have here unto set my hand and caused the seal of the United States to be affixed.

> — President Abraham Lincoln, creating "Fast Day" two months before Gettysburg, (He proclaimed 9 in all!)

An action is virtuous due to its being directed by reason to a noble good. And this is true of fasting. For we fast for three purposes: (1) to restrain the desires of the flesh; (2) to raise the mind to contemplate sublime things; (3) to make satisfaction for our sins. These are good and noble things, and so fasting is virtuous.

> — Thomas Aquinas

A fast is first and foremost personal. It is a fast for the purification of my own body, mind, and soul. The fast is also a heartfelt prayer for purification and strengthening for all those who work beside me in the farm worker movement. The fast is also an act of penance for those in positions of moral authority and for all men and women activists who know what is right and just, who know that they could and should do more. The fast is finally a declaration of non-cooperation with supermarkets who promote and sell and profit from California table grapes... I pray to God that this fast will be a preparation for a multitude of simple deeds for justice. Carried out by men and women whose hearts are focused on the suffering of the poor and who yearn, with us, for a better world. Together, all things are possible.

> — Cesar Chavez

Two things are infinite: the universe and human stupidity; and I'm not sure about the the universe.

> —Albert Einstein, said to fast to think more clearly

Solitude and fasting have from time immemorial been the best-known means of strengthening any meditation whose purpose is to open the door of the unconscious.

> — Carl Jung

Fasting is the strongest appeal to the human being's natural powers of healing and self-rejuvenation, on both a spiritual and corporeal level.

    — Heinz Fahrner, M.D.

Due to the effects of fasting, a fast can help you heal with greater speed; cleanse your liver, kidneys, and colon; purify your blood; help you lose excess weight and water; flush out toxins; clear the eyes and tongue; and cleanse the breath."

    — James F. Balch, M.D

Fasting creates a condition of low concentration of toxic wastes in the circulatory system. This is sensed by the plasma membrane of each cell and each cell will then let go of its load of toxic wastes.

    — Ron Kennedy, M.D.

Fasting is the greatest remedy, the physician within.

    — Paracelsus

Instead of using medicine, fast a day.

    —Plutarch

Who wants to stay strong, healthy and young? Be moderate, exercise the body, breathe pure air, and heal your woes by fasting as well as by medicine.

    — Hippocrates

PERFECT HEALTH! Have you any conception of what the phrase means ? Can you form any image of what would be your feeling if every organ in your body were functioning perfectly? Perhaps you can go back to some day in your youth, when you got up early in the morning and went for a walk, and the spirit of the sunrise got into your blood, and you walked faster, and took deep breaths, and laughed aloud for the sheer happiness of being alive in such a world of beauty. And now you are grown older—and what would you give for the secret of that glorious feeling? What would you say if you were told that you could bring it back and keep it, not only for mornings, but for afternoons and evenings, and not as something accidental and mysterious, but as something which you yourself have created, and of which you are completely master?

This is not an introduction to a new device in patent medicine advertising. I have nothing to sell, and no process patented. It is simply that for ten years I have been studying the ill health of myself and of the men and women around me. And I have found the cause and the remedy. I have not only found good health, but perfect health; I have found a new state of being, a new potentiality of life; a sense of lightness and cleanness and joyfulness, such as I did not know could exist in the human body. The fast is to me the key to eternal youth, the secret of perfect and permanent health. I would not take anything in all the world for my knowledge of it.

     — Upton Sinclair, 1878-1968

Fasting is an institution as old as Adam. It has been resorted to for self-purification or for some ends, noble as well as ignoble. True happiness is impossible without true health. One should eat not in order to please the palate, but just to keep the body going... True health is impossible without the rigid control of the palate… A complete fast is a complete and literal denial of self. It is the truest prayer... A genuine fast cleanses the body, mind and soul. It crucifies the flesh and, to that extent, sets the soul free... My religion teaches me that whenever there is distress which one cannot remove, one must fast and pray... Fasting will bring spiritual rebirth to those of you who cleanse and purify your bodies. The light of the world will illuminate within you when you fast and purify yourself…  When each organ of sense subserves the body and, through the body, the soul, its special relish disappears, and then alone does it begin to function in the way Nature intended it to do.
— Mahatma Gandhi

All any of us are trying to do is precisely that: turn on the light. All the better to see you with, my dear. Christ, Buddha, Mohammed, Moses, Milarepa, and other great ones spent their time in fasting, praying, meditation, and left "maps" of the territory of "God" for all to see and follow in our own way.
— John Lennon, fasting practitioner

In fasting, I am using the same method for physical, mental, and spiritual purification that the greatest spiritual leaders have used throughout the ages.

> — Paul Bragg, co-grandfather (with his senior Bernarr Macfadden) of the American health movement, author of *The Miracle of Fasting*

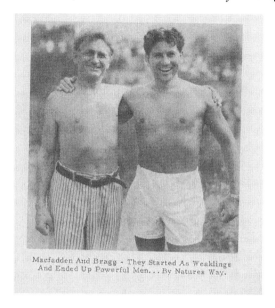

Macfadden And Bragg - They Started As Weaklings And Ended Up Powerful Men...By Natures Way.

As was required of him in Egypt, Pythagoras refused to accept anyone into his school who did not know how to fast. The master was known for his 40 day fasts.

Notable fasters not quoted: Gertrude Stein, Moses, Zoraster, Aristotle, Socrates, Martin Luther, Martin Luther King, Jr., Teresa of Avila, Mother Teresa, Confucius, Lao Tzu, Joan of Arc, Steve Jobs, Nikola Tesla, Thomas Edison, Isaac Newton, Michelangelo ...

## Words of the Day: Pluripotency / Autophagy

You heard me: plural potency. It's when a stem cell can become anything, a modern medical miracle. That's potent indeed, almost the Holy Grail or fountain of youth. Maybe it's the word of the Age. (Entendre intended.)

This story began when the scientists at the University of Southern California Oncology Department were focusing on the tragedy of chemotherapy: the treatment kills more people than the disease, as we all know. The worse part of chemo is how it ravages your white blood cells (and knocks the shit out of your red ones as well), and with a compromised immune system and less capacity, you die from a host of things too easily. Seeking protection from chemotherapy's immunosuppression is paramount.

That's when fellow USC researcher Dr. Victor D. Longo (Edna M. Jones Professor of Gerontology and the Biological Sciences at the USC Davis School of Gerontology and director of the USC Longevity Institute) suggested that some possibilities could come from research he had done on calorie restriction, aging pathways, and fasting to boost white blood cells.

You see, the chemical breakdown and deterioration of our cells is much the same in chemo as it is in aging. The anti-aging research suggested a counter to the cellular horrors of chemo. Dr. Longo reported, "Prolonged fasting also protected against toxicity in a pilot clinical trial in which a small group of

patients fasted for a 72-hour period prior to chemotherapy." —
*Fasting: Molecular Mechanisms and Clinical Applications Cell
Metabolism Review*, Feb 4, 2014 by Valter D. Longo and Mark P.
Mattson.

The results showed that cancer cells are *more vulnerable
to chemotherapy* during the fasting period (and afterwards the
regeneration of healthy cells was significantly improved). The
fasting-induced acute weight loss could easily be restored,
whereas the control group who received chemotherapy
(without fasting) lost weight continuously, without regaining
it. Longo demonstrated "that fasting protects against
chemotherapy-induced side effects and neuronal damages, like
behavioral deficiencies and deficits in motor coordination,
learning, and memory." [Françoise Wilhelmi de Toledo, from
"Eat, Fast, and Live Longer!", his report on the 15th medical
congress of the Medical Association for Fasting and Nutrition
(2013), where Longo received the Maria Buchinger Foundation
Award.]

Co-author Tanya Dorff (assistant professor of clinical
medicine at the USC Norris Comprehensive Cancer Center and
Hospital) concurred, "While chemotherapy saves lives, it
causes significant collateral damage to the immune system.
The results of this study suggest that fasting may mitigate
some of the harmful effects of chemotherapy." And because the
findings are so dramatic, she went on to rightly caution, "More
clinical studies are needed, and any such dietary intervention
should be undertaken only under the guidance of a physician."

Longo took a fresh approach: instead of studying humans or even mammals, he proposed that the benefits of fasting should be able to be seen at a cellular level, not just systemically. Longo examined one-cell creatures enduring a spectrum of fasts and meticulously screened over 6,000 genes in search of aging pathways. As he converted the glucose-feeding-supply to water, the yeasts lived twice as long, *and a host of repair functions were activated*. Yeasts that were fasted were found to be protected from "oxidative insult," or dramatically free from the attacks by free radicals and other agents that damage DNA, thereby inflicting cancer and other ills.

Based on cellular evidence, he studied the effects of fasting on multi-celled creatures, and finding similar benefits, then conducted his own investigation with mice. With an evolutionary tree of precedent (including vibrant survivals from massive doses of chemotherapy), fasts for humans were medically and biochemically observed with the cutting edge of microscopic acuity.

Longo enjoined the National Institute of Health's Longevity Director Mark Mattson for the research and assessment. They reported the amazing efficacy of fasting in countering chemotherapy's ills (larger trials are now in process), **but for those of us who do not have cancer, the data was also clear**: "Clinical and epidemiological data are consistent with an ability of fasting to retard the aging process and associated diseases. Major factors implicated in aging whose generation are accelerated by gluttonous lifestyles and slowed by energy restriction in humans include the following: (1) oxidative damage to proteins, DNA, and lipids; (2) inflammation; (3) accumulation of dysfunctional proteins and organelles; and (4) elevated glucose, insulin, and [timely] IGF-1." They showed how living with just 30% less calories significantly reduced high blood pressure, diabetes, cardiovascular diseases, and obesity, all in one. Instead of 10 different drugs, only 1 health-enhancing procedure would be required. (Bad news for the pharmaceuticals.)

Superpowers.

But before we unpack their findings or get to the bordering-on-miraculous scientific discoveries, we need a review of therapeutic and medical fasting for proper context.

What happens when you fast? Well, as everyone knows, within hours your blood sugar drops; you feel weak, you get a headache, you feel dizzy, you are "hungry", etc. If you are able to eat, you feel better and congratulate yourself on taking good care of your needs. But if you endure the difficulty and don't eat and don't pass out or kill somebody, you set off a host of triggers. Most prominently, when your blood sugar is low enough, the pancreas stops cranking out insulin and from an alternate set of cells secretes the hormone *glucagon*. First of all, the insulin-producing cells are rested when you don't feed, and glucagon prompts the glycogen stores in your liver to convert to glucose. Voila! 'Gas' is flowing again into the billions of mitochondrial factories. (Most people have experienced how

their hunger temporarily disappears during exercise —
because tensing naturally squeezes out the glycogen that is also
stored throughout the musculature.) The first few times you
intentionally endure the suffering of hunger in order to trigger
pancreatic-glucagon-release is quite disconcerting.

Then the really hard part! By the end of the first day or
on the second day, the glycogen stores are emptied and the
body must begin to convert its metabolic avenues from glucose
to fat-burning, or *ketosis*. Most of us haven't used those ketonic
avenues on a regular basis since we were breast-feeding
(though they are ready to go during extreme times we can't get
any food — which is the evolutionary normal). As soon as we
started on solid foods, we converted over to glucose
metabolics, and in modern times where we can get three meals
a day plus snacks, we rarely use the ketonic, fat-burning
avenues.

While it may be very natural, it can be painful to re-
teach the body to make that switch to fats/ketones and the first
few times you re-exercise the pathways of ketosis through
fasting, it can take many unpleasant hours to convert. But if we
do not learn this workout, we inevitably suffer "the diseases of
kings." I prefer fresher, non-meat avenues, but perhaps a good
transition might be to first train the body to adapt to ketosis via
the caveman diet or your favorite ketonic cookbook.

Exercising the glucagon-trigger along with the
reacquiring of ketonic avenues is what I call, "Metabolic
Calisthenics". These capacities are like "muscles" that most
people don't use anymore, and like any muscle or pathway, it

takes more than one or two workouts to gain sufficient strength. Correspondingly, as soon as you build even a little strength in metabolic calisthenics, the exercise becomes relatively easy. In as short as six weeks to six months, depending on a variety of factors, you quickly gain one of the great 'superpowers' of fasting: glucose control.

Because of the glucose-control-strength that comes from metabolic calisthenics, insulin sensitivity is enhanced and that function of the pancreas can rest. The "metabolic syndrome" (the combination of abdominal fat, insulin resistance, elevated triglcerides, and hypertension that elevates the risk of heart disease, type-2 diabetes, stroke, and Alzheimer's Disease) is not ameliorated or helped, but reversed by fasting! The degree to which all aspects of metabolic syndrome is undone is jaw-dropping. Diabetes-2 preset and onset can be reversed by therapeutic (medical), fasting. Blood pressure naturally falls and *hypoglycemia is undone*. Blood sugar problems are the complexes most dramatically impacted and eliminated by therapeutic fasting. The body is no longer subject to blood-sugar highs and lows; your body keeps fuel easily funneled to your cells as needed.

"Prolonged fasting can reverse multiple features of the metabolic syndrome in humans: it enhances insulin sensitivity, stimulates lipolysis, and reduces blood pressure." (*Fasting: Molecular Mechanisms and Clinical Applications Cell Metabolism Review*, Feb 4, 2014 by Valter D. Longo and Mark P. Mattson)

Superpowers!

The second day of a fast can be harder than the first. It's not like a hybrid vehicle, a quick flick of a switch. It usually takes many hours, even all day at first, during which the body is under great stress. In fact, to compensate for low blood sugar on day two, the body even converts a teeny bit of its own muscle mass to sugars (unpleasantly) as the ketonic system ramps up.

Sometime in day three, ketosis has gotten up to speed sufficiently (and continues to gain efficiency for another week!) so that the hunger pains and physiological stresses that accompany fasting begin to fade away. Usually in day three or four (after I crowbar myself out of bed and take a shower), I feel so good, I usually exclaim, "Wow, do I feel great! I'm never going to eat again!"

But in addition to brightening endorphins that also flood the body, other beneficial biochemical cascades are set in motion by the stress of fasting; most prominent of these changes is the growth hormone aptly named "Insulin-like Growth Factor 1". IGF-1 production falls precipitously as our protein intake drops.

To illustrate the role or function of IGF-1, Longo explained that our cellular bodies could be said to have two gears: feeding and healing. When you feed regularly, IGF-1 signals the cellular pace of "go-go", and this drives whole chains of enzymes and stress hormones, as well as much quicker cell division. But if you always drive your car, Longo explains, and never take it in for service or cleaning, it simply won't last as long, or be as efficient [or smell as well].

When your IGF-1 level drops from a variety of fasting modalities, hunger causes the cells to shift gears and go into self-service, repair, balance, and clean mode. Noteworthy in this repair and refresh mode is how your body attends to errors in your DNA. The impact of this is huge.

For emphasis, Longo studied hundreds of people in an extended large family in Ecuador who suffered from Laron syndrome, a congenital condition where receptors of growth hormone production are impaired, greatly reducing regular IGF-1 production. Although they were all quite short in stature (three-foot adults were common), there is zero history of cancer, diabetes and cardiovascular disease! — despite their terrible habits, including overeating and tobacco consumption. They even relished in their intoxications and indulgences, knowing they would never get the common diseases of aging.

While "go-go" cellular metabolism accomplishes much growth in a go-go-go world, IGF-1 directly correlates to aging, insulin resistance and tumor progression. A variety of diets and partial fasting programs lower IGF-1, lowering cancer and cardiovascular possibilities from forty to eighty percent.

While there are levels of benefit with varying levels of fasting, Longo showed that most of the advantages are inherited with minimal programs! All you have to do is adapt to just about any of the 10,000 ways to do so, from Lent fasts, Ramadan, and Calorie Restriction to the currently "popular" Michael Mosley's 5-2 diet (eat like you want for five days a wek, on two days keep the calories below approximately 500).

The key is that you learn to regularly endure, sustain, and even enjoy the temporary discomfort of **chosen hunger**.

As IGF-1 and glucose levels drop, your cellular division slows greatly, and your cells go into full repair mode — making sure they are in the cleanest, best shape possible. From the cell wall to the nucleus and mitochondrial DNA, your cells repair and refresh. This cellular care-mode increases their lifespan by as much as 40% (hint-hint) and all but eliminates the errors that instigate the unrestricted growth of cancer.

Anti-cancer, longer life: Superpowers.

Once you adapt to some sort of regular fasting and receive significant anti-cancer, anti-diabetes, anti-cardiovascular resistance (~six months to two years depending on your health), you come to sufficient strength to properly go deeper and longer. Deeper benefits can be harvested, but the foundation must be there. Check with your doctor, of course, to make sure there is no pressing issue you should take into account, then slowly build up to foundational ease with a modified, intermittent fasting program (see below). Again, this foundation could take six weeks to twenty-four months. But when ease and understanding are present, deep benefits will be easily gained.

The 15th medical congress of the Medical Association for Fasting and Nutrition took place on June 29–30, 2013 in Überlingen, Germany and emphasized modified fasts and their benefits thusly: "Nowadays, fasting-mimicking and enhancing diets (FMED) are being developed in order to motivate people to fast without having to completely renounce food. Although this may seem contradicting, these low-calorie diets with a special composition have some of the metabolic and neurohormonal effects of fasting, like diminishing fat mass, enhancing insulin sensitivity, boosting stem cells, and reducing activity of some aging pathways. They can of course not replace the holistic effects of a whole fasting process, but could help people maintaining the good results on the long run."

### Word of the Day #2: Autophagy

As day two kicks into gear and you have exhausted digestive sugars, muscular glucose, and the liver stores as well, the glucagon signals the cells to STOP all mitosis and stimulates the formation of **lysosomes** in the cells' cytoplasm. The creation of these 'garbage disposal' organelles puts the processes of **autophagy** into high gear.

Autophagy is from the Greek, for 'self-eating', and the recent breakthroughs in the study of autophagy has been heralded as "A New Field of Medicine". Autophagy, our second "word of the day", is so important to the study of fasting, that it is worthy of a bit of study and elaboration.

In 1949, Christian de Duve, the chairman of the Laboratory of Physiological Chemistry at the Catholic University of Louvain in Belgium, led a team to study the cellular enzymes in the liver in response to glucose-triggered insulin and the series of enzymes surrounding this. They then followed those sames cells in response to glucose-low glucagon. (De Duve coined the name *glucagon* in 1951.) In response to stresses, cells created different "saclike structures surrounded by a membrane" and contained a host of enzymes, depending on the kind of stress the cell was managing. He called these sacs "lysosomes" (Greek for 'loosening' or 'dissolving' 'bodies'). Research into these lysosomes revealed that they contain hydrolytic, 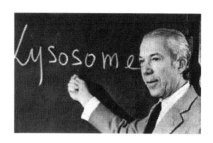 digestive-like enzymes that can break down *any* kind of biomolecule. Over the decades it would become clear that these sacs served a host of functions: energy, remodeling proteins, defense, but most obvious of all, it was certainly a garbage disposal. Somehow, damaged or dying cell parts, unwanted enzymes, and fats would be eaten by these sacs and then spit out streams of refreshed proteins for building and energy for cellular functions.

In 1963, de Duve coined the term "autophagy", Greek for "self-eating", to describe the "re-utilization of cellular materials," and "disposal of organelles". Along with two others, he won the Nobel prize in 1974, for "their discoveries concerning the structural and functional organization of the cell".

Autophagy is now known as a normal part of a cell's lifespan. Individual cells can "eat" parts of themselves, especially old or damaged parts, and recycle the material to help keep themselves healthy. (Virus and bacteria are also disposed of in the lysosomes by the same autophagic process.)

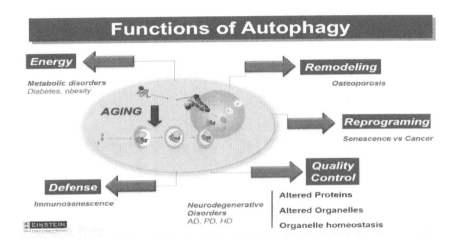

By shedding damaged or dying parts inside the cell, the cell has a new resource from which to repair itself and keep itself running. If this function is robust, the quality and length of life is enlarged. The process is seen to be awry in cancer, infectious diseases, immunological diseases and neurodegenerative disorders. Because of the repair-and-refresh functions of autophagy, disruption of these functions play a significant role in the aging process.

A dysfunctional autophagy process has also been linked to Type 2 diabetes and other genetic diseases. In particular, it may play an important role in two distinct disease types that are difficult to treat and mysterious in origin: cancer and neurodegenerative disease.

Yoshinori Ohsumi, a Japanese cell biologist, was awarded the 2016 Nobel Prize in Physiology or Medicine for his discoveries on the genetics that guide autophagy.

"Autophagy was kind of a sleepy backwater of a research topic," says biochemist Michael Hall of the University of Basel in Switzerland. "It was basically considered the garbage-disposal system of the cell — just bulk, non-specific degradation of junk."

Dr. David H. Perlmutter, dean of the School of Medicine at Washington University in St. Louis, said Dr. Ohsumi's work opened a field that has now exploded, with implications that are "the stuff of science fiction." If the autophagy system is knocked out, he said, *the result is premature aging, with ailments like cardiovascular disease, skeletal weakness, glucose intolerance and cognitive decline.* Now drugs that stimulate this system are being studied. "If you take a drug and stimulate the system, you will make the organism live longer in a cancer-free way," he said. Kay F. Macleod, a cancer researcher at the University of Chicago, added, "It is super exciting that autophagy has been recognized in and of itself."

When autophagy starts to slow down or stop functioning properly, the cell can no longer destroy its abnormal proteins, old cell structures and invasive germs. Disruptions in autophagy have also been linked to Parkinson's disease, type 2 diabetes and other disorders — and research is ongoing to develop drugs that can affect the process. In Parkinson's, scientists have linked dysfunctional autophagy processes to the accumulation of Lewy bodies.

In the same way, amyloid plaques, another kind of damaging protein, may also accumulate if the autophagy process breaks down. Researchers suspect Amyloid plaques cause Alzheimer's disease.

Jay Debnath, a professor of pathology at the University of California, San Francisco, who is using Ohsumi's discoveries to develop breast cancer treatments, explained that this could be because brain cells have stopped "eating" abnormal 'garbage' proteins.

Therapies to help re-start the autophagy process may help cells clear the toxic proteins that are inhibiting their function. For instance, in a small phase 1 trial, people with Parkinson's disease and Lewy body dementia who received a small, daily dose of an FDA-approved leukemia drug that happens to promote autophagy experienced improvements in motor skills and cognition over six months.

In fact, fasting (which raises glucagon) naturally provides the greatest known boost to autophagy. Fasting, of course, is far more beneficial than just stimulating autophagy. It does two good things. By stimulating autophagy, we are clearing out all our old, junky proteins and cellular parts. At the same time, fasting also stimulates growth hormone, which tells our body to start producing some new snazzy parts for the body. We truly give our bodies a complete renovation.

On day three, you can feel a new level of autophagy kick into high gear called *autolysis*. You not only eat intra-cellular garbage and damage, you start actively eating other cells. Ah, here's where nature shows off its innate intelligence. For the proteins and energy we still require, your body doesn't just start eating anything or everything, but naturally starts cleaning house. Cells that are damaged or compromised in any way in all systems are harvested. Thus it is said that the autolysis and autophagy of fasting provides an "operation without surgery".

For the first two days, the linings of your stomach and intestines are cleansed as the oldest and damaged cells from your throat through your large intestine are consumed. Your alimentary canal is thoroughly rested, refreshed, and renewed.

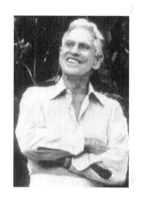

Eating away your diseased, inflamed, and damaged sections (in every system) is another empowerment that comes from fasting (details to follow). As master-faster Paul Bragg, (my first inspiration 41 years ago) used to *brag* in his sixties and seventies, "I have an ageless, tireless, painless body."

Superpowers.

In addition to intestinal cleaning, our bodies naturally consume a most available protein — the germ fighters just floating around through the bloodstream: the white-blood cells or leukocytes. First your body eats all the damaged leukocytes as well as those memory T-cells that are 'saturated' (and thus inefficient in their war on new germs). After fasting for four days, your white blood cell count is cut in half!

Upon feeding again, your white blood cell count normalizes (and the red blood cells get a normalizing and refreshing boost as well). Longo and his team asked, "Where did those extra blood cells suddenly come from?" Only a tiny fraction could be there from natural cell production in the marrow.

Now here's where it gets interesting. In addition to lower levels of IGF-1, prolonged fasting reduces an enzyme central to the regulation of glucose and lipids called *protein kinase A* or PKA for short. PKA is directly linked to longevity and *the regulation of stem-cell self-renewal: pluripotency*, the ability for a cell to develop into any thing the body needs.

"PKA is the key gene that needs to shut down in order for these stem cells to switch into regenerative mode. It gives the okay for stem cells to go ahead and begin proliferating and rebuild the entire system," explained Doctor Longo. "And the good news is that the body got rid of the parts of the system that might be damaged or old, the inefficient parts, during the fasting... We could not predict that prolonged fasting would have such a remarkable effect in promoting

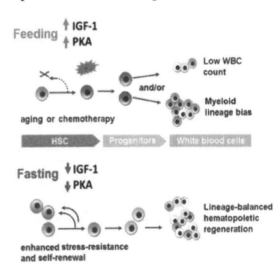

stem cell-based regeneration of the hematopoietic system [blood stem cells]... Now, if you start with a system heavily damaged by chemotherapy or aging, fasting cycles can generate, literally, a new immune system."

Superpower bam!

Valter Longo and The National Institute of Health's Director of Longevity Mark Mattson published their findings on pluripotency as "Fasting: Molecular Mechanisms and Clinical Applications" in the *Cell Stem Cell* (Vol. 14 Issue 6 June 2014, pp. 810-823). They showed that fasting was far more efficacious than any anti-chemo drug available and its application to wide variety of diseases was highly noteworthy. Because of the highly technical language in that publication, an introductory overview of it can be found in the USC Keck School of Medicine overview article (June 10, 2014): "Fasting triggers stem cell regeneration of damaged old immune system." (*Graphs above and below from said article.*)

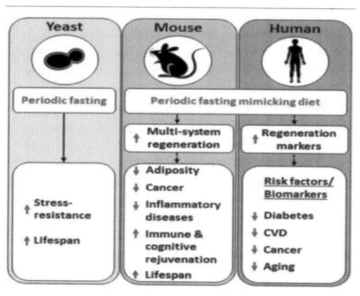

Some gifts just keep on giving: The findings of regeneration were not limited to the immune system and the red-blood cells. The National Institute of Health was particularly impressed with how neural networks showed vigorous cellular regeneration — actual new brain cells, in response to the stress of fasting. "If you can't find food, you better enlarge your brain!"

[See the NIH's Longevity director, Mark Mattson, speak of this and the implications and findings in the areas of Alzheimer's, Parkinson's and Huntington's diseases at https://www.youtube.com/watch?v=4UkZAwKoCP8]

Superpowers.

Longo and his fellows also presented research that showed a dramatic reduction in overall inflammation during fasting. Evidence suggested that if you fast seven to eleven days, you can even base a cure for rheumatoid arthritis, providing you eliminated meat in the diet upon re-feeding.

The medical applications of therapeutic fasting, based on new evidence, are pan-systemic, with particular application in fighting cancer, cardio-vascular disease, neural networks (including Alzheimer's, Parkinson's, and Huntington's diseases), inflammatory issues, and aging. Many studies confirm it, but a most poignant (and inadvertant) one is that lifespan increased by 6 years in the U.S.A. during the worst of the Great Depression.

We need to understand that "Metabolic Calisthenics" is most unpleasant at first, but this level of difficulty "quickly" abates and only occasional discomfort remains (along with a plethora of wonderful visitations). Adapting to our alternative energy power is a workout, and like most workouts, it is quite different two months into it as it was the beginning. In fact, Longo and his team showed evidence that the shift in metabolic avenues could normalize after only six weeks of off and on fasting.

"Once you get used to it, it's not a big deal," said Dr. Mattson, chief of the National Institute of Health's laboratory of neurosciences. "It's just a matter of getting adapted to it… If you've been sedentary for years and then you go out and try to run five miles, you're not going to feel very good until you get in shape," he said. " It's not going to be a smooth transition right away."

Correlations to this metabolic-pathways re-wiring are found in programs designed for recovery from addictions. Going to a recovery *weekend* is most likely not going to change your life. But if you can keep with the program and stay sober for six weeks, new metabolic and biochemical pathways to satisfaction can appear and the struggle is more easily managed.

Fasting programs have long trumpeted the superpower of detoxification and cleansing. For good reason. When the body's processes of assimilation and elimination are relieved of the assimilation, the body's energy for elimination is greatly enhanced and a deep cleaning takes place. As the six-times New York Times best-selling author Dr. Joel Fuhrman emphasizes, "The fast does not merely detoxify; it also breaks down superfluous tissue - fat, abnormal cells, atheromatous plaque [arterial blockage], and tumors--and releases diseased tissues and their cellular products into the circulation for elimination. Toxic or unwanted materials circulate in our bloodstream and lymphatic tissues, and are deposited in and released from our fat stores and other tissues. An important element of fasting detoxification is mobilizing the toxins from their storage areas."

Cleanliness is next to godliness indeed, as the cleansing of fasting makes for room for *native radiance*, true health.

We must come to see the scientific and medical value in the opposite of go-go-go and be rested, repaired, and refreshed. Or are we addicted to dependency or unwilling to pay for our own experience? The dues are steep at first, no doubt, but the benefits are mountainous with plural potencies and authentic vistas. So in addition to medical and biological superpowers, I would be remiss if I failed to re-emphasize that fasting has long been valued for its evocative and spiritual blessings. Superpowers indeed, and in truth.

While the great spiritual teachers have praised fasting, as seen in the first chapter, "A World of Praise for Fasting", let me end with a modern great. When asked where he got his energy while walking across India, Gandhi quipped Socratic-ly, "From fasting!" He went on to say, "The light of the world will illuminate within you when you fast and purify yourself. What the eyes are to the outward vision, fasting is to the inward."

# My Dietary Journey to Optimal Nutrition
# and Bodily Wisdom

I started making my own money at 5 years of age, selling pencils door-to-door. One for 2¢, two for a nickel (cute mistake); I raked it in. I used the money to buy candy… which I proceeded to eat in lots for the next decade and a half. When I was finally living on my own, the first thing I bought with my first paycheck was a case of Snickers.

Other than my sugar addiction, I ate pretty well for a kid in the South in the fifties and sixties; I had plenty of southern veggies and iceberg lettuce along with my meats and fast food. My dad was from Puerto Rico, so we ate a lot of rice and beans, too (thank god). Bodily, I was very athletic: climbing, swimming, diving, and developing the art of rope-swinging (go figure). On the down-side, I sustained a few severe head injuries. The upside is that I set records in grade school and high school for sit-ups, push-ups and pull-ups.

In college, I consumed my share of sixties intoxicants and celebrated. I left school and lived on a remote farm near the Appalachians (no electricity or running water). I enjoyed the freshest of foods and rugged living for over two years. I was super-healthy and weighed 135 pounds.

But slaughtering and growing my own food taught me a few things. Freshness of food and robustness of life are related; bringing out the best tastes and nutrition in foods is a great art; and despite some nutritional advantages of meat, I didn't like killing animals for my food.

I became a vegetarian and moved back to Nashville. I
ate a banana split every night instead of meat. Slowly, I began
passing out when getting out of bed in the morning. Then,
getting out of a chair would usually make me dizzy. Between
the lack of good nutrition and over-use of sugar, I had
developed a severe shortage of the enzyme that co-oxidizes
glucose, thiamin, or vitamin B-1, "the morale vitamin". (It also
seemed to me that my heriditary low-blood pressure combined
with the multiple head wounds guided my passings into
unconsciousness.) I have blacked-out hundreds of times.

Now the first
"miracle story". In
August 1975, *People*
magazine ran an article
on Paul Bragg's 94th
birthday. Now for
those of you who do
not know of Paul
Bragg, let me just say
that Paul Bragg is the
one of the grandfathers
of the American health
movement. He was a
phenomena. The
picture in People said it
all: he looked 56, not
94, and was positively

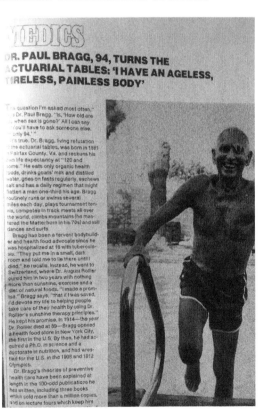

**MEDICS**

**DR. PAUL BRAGG, 94, TURNS THE ACTUARIAL TABLES: 'I HAVE AN AGELESS, TIRELESS, PAINLESS BODY'**

The question I'm asked most often," says Dr. Paul Bragg, "is, 'How old are you when sex is gone?' All I can say is you'll have to ask someone else. I'm only 94.' "

It's true. Dr. Bragg, living refutation of the actuarial tables, was born in 1881 in Fairfax County, Va. and reckons his own life expectancy at "120 and some." He eats only organic health foods, drinks goats' milk and distilled water, goes on fasts regularly, eschews salt and has a daily regimen that might flatten a man one-third his age. Bragg routinely runs or swims several miles each day, plays tournament tennis, competes in track meets all over the world, climbs mountains (he mastered the Matterhorn in his 70s) and still dances and surfs.

Bragg has been a fervent bodybuilder and health food advocate since he was hospitalized at 16 with tuberculosis. "They put me in a small, dark room and told me to lie there until I died," he recalls. Instead, he went to Switzerland, where Dr. August Rollier cured him in two years with nothing more than sunshine, exercise and a diet of natural foods. "I made a promise," Bragg says, "that if I was saved, I'd devote my life to helping people take care of their health by using Dr. Rollier's sunshine therapy principles." He kept his promise. In 1914—the year Dr. Rollier died at 89—Bragg opened a health food store in New York City, the first in the U.S. By then, he had acquired a Ph.D. in science and a doctorate in nutrition, and had wrestled for the U.S. in the 1908 and 1912 Olympics.

Dr. Bragg's theories of preventive health care have been explained at length in the 100-odd publications he has written, including three books, which sold more than a million copies, and on lecture tours which keep him

46

radiant (later I found out that he was in fact 79, a self-promoter's long-lived lie). In any case, I looked at him and said, "Whatever that guy's doing, I'm gonna try it." He was the demonstration of health—and fortunately, was an enthusiastic prophet of how to follow him.

Following Paul Bragg's recommendations, the first thing I added to my diet was nutritional yeast, a super-food rich in B vitamins. Instantly, my regular black-outs were almost eliminated and my over-all energy level rocketed. I was impressed. The immensity of the change prompted me to pose a question to myself: If the addition of this *one thing* to my diet made this much change, how good can you feel? **Really, how good can you feel?**

Attending first to the body, I began a three-year study of nutrition. In addition to Bragg, I read volumes — from Adelle Davis to college texts on nutrition. My favorite book was *The Nutrition Almanac*, with a vast Table of Food Composition. But in addition to continuous book learning, I kept a health diary and began a serious 'data diving' investigation.

In my health diary, I recorded everything I ate, when, how I felt, and noted exercise patterns. At the end of every week, I tabulated and evaluated. I calculated all crucial (to me) categories, how much calcium, protein, vitamins, magnesium, sodium, iodine, etc. etc., I had consumed. I noted balances (sodium-potassium, protein-carbohydrates, calcium-magnesium, etc.). I adjusted my diet accordingly. Over a few months, I memorized the *Table of Food Composition* as it related to my diet. For three years, I kept a constant eye to optimize my nutritional profiles and maximize my capacity for energy and harmony.

Reading a variety of nutrition books, I quickly noted widespread differences of opinion. For instance, some books favored 60+ grams of protein daily, others said 10! So I experimented: for two-month segments I ate 35 concentrated grams of protein daily, then 25, then 15, then 10, back to 15 and finally decided my optimum was in the 20 gms/day neighborhood, adjusting slightly lower to the warmer seasons. I did not lose sight of my original enquiry: how good can you feel? For dedicated detail to optimizing every kind of dietary nuance obviously occurred within a greater picture of freeing feeling — which intermeshed with exercise and psychology.

At the end of the third year of this enquiry and experimentation, my health program looked like this: I squeezed a large glass of orange juice for breakfast, and for lunch and dinner I had a hearty salad (with nuts, seeds, yeast, sprouted legumes, and nutritionally rich dressings); I swam three miles a week, sauna-ed twice a week, I ran 38 miles a week, and I followed Paul Bragg's "secret": I fasted one day a week, three days a month and one week every year.

While the benefits of fasting are many, there is one potency that is generally unsung: the overall capacity to manage glucose and energy levels.

When your blood sugar drops, your body signals the mind to think, "I'm hungry." You eat something, your blood sugar goes back up, you feel better, and you congratulate yourself on taking care of yourself. But this glucose management system traps you in a roller coaster of insulin and glucose levels, slowly robs you of overall energy, exhausts your pancreas, and usually fosters overweight conditions, including diabetes 2.

Through a variety of modes of fasting, we can learn to keep our energy levels high, even though metabolics is supposedly an "involuntary" process. To conceive of how this is possible, imagine a set of proverbial twins: one runs daily, the other is far more sedentary. Now put them both into a sauna. Mr. Or Ms Studness relaxes and enjoys the sweat; Mr./Ms. Officeperson experiences difficulty. Exercise-Person has learned to sweat and gain some control of an involuntary process. This sweating analogy conveys the idea that we can gain similar capacity to keep our metabolic levels high.

Instead of automatically eating, we slowly learn to endure more and more hunger until the blood sugar comes back up (yes, you will probably get irritable and maybe a bit crazy). In doing so, we exercise those pancreatic and metabolic processes that turn glycogen into glucose, then fats into fuel. Bragg's system of regular fasting exercised my metabolic capacities and allowed me to take my overall dynamism to a new level.

Maintaining a fasting yoga, my energy level was off the charts, let me Bragg. Ripples of energy, swells of potency, and bubbles of health were my constant experience. I only weighed 9 pounds less than my peak (135-9=126). Twenty-five years old,

I ran a hardware store, opened a highly successful natural foods restaurant (I needed a place to go out), I taught optimal nutrition-"cooking" class at a local college, I bought an old church (1910) and renovated it for my home. I traveled; I continued my studies of nutrition, athletics, philosophy, and spirituality. I had more energy than most 20 people combined.

By living with a rigorous discipline, I observed key issues about why people eat the way they do:

**1. Most people eat for balance.** No matter how you're feeling, a sit-down meal will help you feel better. Obviously, blood sugar is brought up and electrolytic balances are enhanced— and rest provides much relief and refreshment.

**2. People eat for a pleasurable sense of connectedness**. In a positive light, the sharing of food enhances the sense of community, companionship, and communion. Unhealthy versions of this need can be seen when one is suffering, a morsel of food gives a moment of pleasure. If one is lonely, oral satisfaction feels something like love. Along these lines, Adi Da inspired a cookie shoppe in the 1980's and wrote the following meditation for it.

> *A man does not eat a cookie because he is hungry; a man eats a cookie because he is suffering and needs a small moment of happiness.*
> *A woman does not eat a cookie because she likes sweets; a woman eats a cookie because she is lonely and needs love. Children do not eat cookies because they are suffering or because they are lonely; children eat cookies because they are hungry and like sweets. Only happiness and love and sweetness can satisfy a man, a woman, and a child.*

**3. Coping with stress**. Food helps in many ways to cope with and burn through difficulties in life.

**4**. While other reasons drive people to eat the way they do, **nutritional needs are usually the last thing** to be considered.

*So if one can attend to the sense of balance in one's life, minimize stress, and cultivate one's innate sense of connectedness and trust, then the urges that drive one to eat in an unhealthy manner are diminished.* Then one's real nutritional needs can be optimized. Therefore, we learn to maximize the sense of balance in life, and cultivate connectedness, community, and communion. By such holistic dedication, we will deepen our fundamental trust, and thereby our dietary urges normalize.

At this time in 1977, my body felt absolutely pure, with maximum conduction of bodily energy. I lived in an ascended state, and I had become wealthy. My enquiry, 'how good can you feel?' continued however, because what then stood out were the limitations in feeling. My studies had always included spirituality, philosophy, and religion and now these were paramount. I told my sister, "Ain't no more dirt in my body, whatever is dirty comes out of my mouth, not into it." I studied constantly, but after reading the works of Avatara Adi Da for a couple of years, I sold everything I owned (1978) and lived as a religious renunciate for a decade.

In the ashram/community, I was already living the strict dietary conditions, and I'm sure I was quite obnoxious. But after a year, my teacher noted that a few people in the ashram were living the (conventionally) strict diet as their own little indulgence.

In a similar light, Adi Da critiqued the whole faux-spiritual approach to fasting as in fact furthering vital obsession. *"In most traditional cultures, the fast from gross foods has always been accompanied by intensified moral consideration and/or religious and spiritual practice. For centuries the Jews have fasted on many holy days each year, including their annual 'Day of Atonement.' The Chinese have traditionally fasted and abstained from sexual intercourse before the first spring plowing and sowing of seeds. Christians, Muslims, Buddhists, and men and women of other faiths have practiced fasting as a periodic adjunct to their religious practices. And monks and spiritual aspirants the world over, from Hindu yogis to American Indian medicine men, have used fasting and other means of bodily purification to serve their spiritual awakening or understanding.*

*"Such traditional practices are honorable and authentic; they have moral value for the practitioner. But for many people, "spiritual" fasting is mere self-indulgence. Some people like to fast because they like the sensation created when the vital energy normally used in the food process rises from the lower physical functions and creates a sensation of intensified energy in the whole body. Thus, you may feel euphoric while fasting—but you may also feel somewhat imbalanced emotionally, particularly if the body is relatively toxic. When the physical dimension is brought to rest by fasting and the vital energy is not being used physically, the excess vital energy reflects itself in the emotonal being. Thus, prolonged fasting and*

*improper diet actually exaggerate the emotional being and create a kind of anarchy among body, emotions, and mind.*

*"Therefore, fasting for long periods for spiritual purposes is futile and deluding. It is not really spiritual, even though it creates qualities that people think are spiritual by exaggerating the vital energy and allowing it to overwhelm the psychic or emotional being.*

*"True religious and spiritual life is a conscious affair that transcends all the functions of the lower life. No form of self-conscious working on the mind, the emotional life, or the vital and physical life can truly affect one's religious and spiritual life. At best it can serve moral "repentance" or reconsideration of one's action, and it can be combined with a period of intensified devotional or meditative practice."*

Adi Da had me and a few others take on a "horse-gut" diet: nothing raw, 5-7 meals daily, with emphasis on foods such as potatoes and peanut butter! I don't remember if I gained 9 pounds in 7 days or 7 pounds in 9 days. I am not exaggerating when I state that it was one of the hardest things I ever did.

I was, in fact, shocked at the profundity of the lesson my beloved Adi Da was giving me. First, I noticed how more incarnate I was (of course), but it shattered an idealism I implicitly and deeply held. You see, just as Adi Da critiqued, super-pure diet gives similar sensations and avenues of feeling as some intoxicants and yogic practices: there is a definite feeling that God is sublimely within and subtly up. (Leading to delusions.) Suddenly I felt the difference: God is as much down as up; in fact, love is more here than within. I abandoned my super-purity and continued to gain weight, although I still ate very well, by common standards.

After ten years, I left the formal confines of the ashram life, gained some more weight, got married, gained more weight, had two kids, gained more weight (there's a theme here), went back to school full-time (while maintaining full-time employment), gained even more. I abandoned my fasting practices for too long. Food as a stress management tool got me.

Then, the fateful day came, ten years ago: June 11th, 2006, when I turned in my last thesis, "An Integral Approach to Affective Education" (for my Master's degree in the Arts of Teaching). I was 183 pounds, my cholesterol was 343, and I was ready to resume my practices of optimal nutrition.

The next day I fasted, intending to go several days, but at the day's end, I decided to eat a salad, "to clean out and balance." I began anew the next day, but at day's end, I decided to have an evening salad again. The next day remained the same. I liked the rhythm so much I decided to try it out as a general model. A decade later, this "perpetual Ramadan" continues to be my dietary pattern. Five or six days a week, I do what is called "a modified fast".

The great Bernarr MacFadden, co-grandfather of the American health movement, also promoted this approach and pointed to the foundations of Western history to support it. "During the zenith period of Grecian and Roman civilization monogamy was not half as firmly established as the rule that a health-loving man should content himself with one meal a day, and never eat till he had leisure to digest, that is, not till the day's work was wholly done.

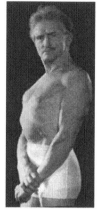

"For more than a thousand years, the one-meal plan was the established rule among the civilized nations inhabiting the coast-lands of the Mediterranean."

This is not entirely true for we have several mentions of pancakes and figs upon rising in *The Illiad*, but this was considered a snack, not a meal. A piece of fruit midday was also not considered a meal, yet common. The eating cycle was indeed centered and heavily weighted in the evening meal.

Herodotus reported that as the vast armies of Persia went through the land, the conquered took heart that the masses of men as well as the Monarch and courtiers only ate one meal at the end of the day. The Jews from Moses until Jesus ate but one meal a day. (They sometimes added a lunch of fruit.) The Hebrew scripture echoes this practice: "Woe unto the nation whose princes eat in the morning."

One modified fast has shown surprising efficacy in developing the benefits and strengths of fasting. Simply make an 8-hour span between meals (optimized at 11am to 7 pm).

Instead of weekly 36-hour fasts, I now do five 24-hour modified fasts a week (I have 1/3 gallon or 125ml of tea in the morning with a piece of dry toast, and nothing but water until dinner). Most days a week, I am very hungry for hours. I have gained new understandings, power, and enjoyment by entering into regular, sustained hunger. I enjoy many of the benefits of more extreme fasting or calorie restriction, but in a fashion that I enjoy (as a four-decades faster). In addition to my almost daily fasts, I usually engage two or three 4-6 day fasts a year, although sometimes I keep going because it's feeling so, so fine. Because I am experienced, I usually don't change anything else about my life while fasting: I work as a school teacher, I hike, I cook for my family, although I do rest more.

Calorie restriction is the only thing repeatedly proven to significantly lengthen life spans, but reducing calories is not the point: it should merely be the <u>effect</u> when nutrition is optimized. *The waist is a terrible thing to mind.* Rather, put your mind on radiant health, not losing weight. Don't worry about reducing calories; put your attention on optimal nutrition. Naturally, this will have growing amounts of the freshest of foods. Cooking will be slowly minimized, and there will be less and less room for calories. And don't worry: celebration and flexibility are not only possible, they are required... so says Mr. Snickers-man. Or in the words of my beloved Adi Da, "Discipline without celebration is obnoxious."

I have crafted my diet as my personal and present response to food and energy. I break any rule anytime (though not very often). When I am comforting myself, I eat sweets at night (usually my own stevia-sweetened granola, an apple/berries and half a cup of non-fat yogurt), and when I go to a party, I may go wild. I call my approach, "flexitarianism". When I go to a Thanksgiving celebration, I eat turkey, all the

trimmings, and every dessert, but usually, it's just a salad+.
[Hearty greens, cabbage and/or sunflower sprouts, chopped
carrot, purple onion, a bit of quinoa or brown rice with yeast
flakes and seeds/nuts with a nutritionally rich dressing.
Dressing: tofu with olive oil, water, much garlic, teaspoon of
miso, sunflower seeds, squeeze of lemon, touch of balsamic,
piece of purple onion, and usually a bit of brown rice. To
thicken, I add nutritional yeast.]

    Instead of having rules to follow, I keep my eye on two
dials: cut and comfort. Discipline and ease. Instead of mental
abstractions, I feel to keep both principles active. Sometimes,
"cut" is strong and I eat fewer sweets and take on more fasts
and fresher foods, and sometimes "comfort" is strong, and I eat
more or anything. Slow but slow is my motto, and I dance to
life's two-step. Accepting the myriad of myself and exercising
the pleasures of celebration and discipline, I let go in oceanic
Life-Light. How good can you feel? Diet and health are
foundational, but free feeling is paramount.

## The Easy Way and the Hard Way

The great thing about learning to fast is that you can start out easy. Keep in mind that hunger is the trigger that sets off the change in your biochemistry. Learning to tolerate and value hunger *is* the dance, the yoga. Everyone makes the error that the craving you feel when you first cease eating will multiply intolerably. In fact, it builds to the needed intensity to set off a new series of biochemical cascades, then fades. Hunger comes and goes, and with every round, it is less compelling. In fact, appetite all but goes away. You will quickly come to appreciate chosen hunger's dance and power.

Exercise the metabolic calisthenics however you want; just do it for at least six months. I tell people to start by simply stretching the time between meals one day a week (I like Thursdays), until you can skip a meal with relative ease. Once skipping one meal is relatively easy, go for two, then after a couple of months or so, see if you can do all day and just eat a hearty salad for dinner (keep it under 500 calories for the day).

After ~three months of gaining strength in chosen hunger, see if you can skip that final meal! Going to bed hungry that first, full-day fast is most definitely difficult. Go as slowly as you want. Quit whenever you want, fail freely. Cheat whenever you need, judge not; take a year or two, just keep working it. "Slow but slow" is my motto (credit to Paul Hughes, who also quipped, "Work is aptly named.")

The great Bernarr MacFadden agreed. "Unquestionably it would be better in experimenting with fasting to start by fasting one meal or say one day at a time. The result of this will give you confidence in its benefits, then you can gradually advance into a full-fledged convert. The principal result of value in such a conversion will be from that day forward absolute independence of all advisers, medical or otherwise, upon an ailment of any kind that attacks you. Fasting will be at once the principal **part** of your self-treatment, and forever thereafter your stomach will be free from the drug habit, for if you expect to retain the slightest respect for yourself you must first learn to respect your stomach." [This exaggeration is based on partial knowledge and 19th century medicine, but the point remains the same.]

Ramadan also accomplishes much as well; many programs do, like simple calorie restriction (which I consider more difficult, but many people like the "CR way"). Please consider a six-month initial engagement with whatever plan(s) you choose; just let your body come to a kind of peace with the sensation of **chosen hunger**. After six weeks, it will be easier, but after six-months, a real strength grounds your new intelligence.

People tell me all the time, "Oh I could never fast!" and then inevitably explain their syndrome (which is usually cured by fasting). I reply that it just like learning to run a marathon. At first, most think, "Oh I could never do that." But can you walk around the block once? If you take it on, you'll be up to twice around the block before long, and if you keep it up, before you know it, the pleasure of running empowers you.

After many rounds of fasting, you gain the simple self-understanding of how flimsy the mind's blabber can be. You learn the lesson of discipline: Tell the blabbing thoughts to mind their own business and instead attend to the greater intelligence, beyond this moment's urgency. After getting a couple of years of regular fasting under your belt (so to speak), and you are harvesting the clear mind of discipline, I recommend a much more difficult approach to prolonged fasting *for those so inclined*.

Plan nothing except your last days of eating. Make sure you eat plenty of raw veggies and salad, maximizing freshness. Then just stop eating. See what you think you need. If you think that you should stop your fast after 6 hours, do so. If you think you should have or have not a little soymilk in your tea, that's good. If you think fasting is best with juices, exactly. If you think you should do only water, terrific. In other words, feel. With a history and foundation of discipline, you can let feeling be your guide. No judgments, feel. No plan. Feel. You can fast 10,000 ways.

I have never been to a fasting clinic or even stopped working when I fast. Two weeks of teaching elementary school while not eating can be easy or quite difficult (usually depending on the kids!) I like to fast and hike. There is even a German word "fastenwandern", which means hiking and fasting together. So it's not a crazy as it sounds.

When I start a fast, I have an inkling that I'd like it to be a moderate (two-four days) or prolonged fast. But generally there is no goal, for a goal can obscure one's feeling. I often have an idea of how long I might fast, but live free to feel.

Two difficult things about longer fasts stand out for me. Without the heat-generation of digestion going on, it is hard to stay warm while sleeping. I'll have flannel sheets, cotton blanket, two comforters and a cover in the spring and summer when I'm fasting. My other difficulty is getting up in the morning. I sleep hard and deep anyway, but upon waking in a long fast, I am slammed to the bed. *Every* morning I think, "Oh shit, I feel like I just got run over; I'm gonna eat today." Sitting upright to get my blood pressure up before standing, I stagger to the shower. After I finish with cold water, I realize again how the mind works and shine into the day.

Every morning, fasting or not, I drink my large volume of tea. Flush, flush, flush is the body's natural way to clean itself. On day one of a fast, I drop the toast. Starting day two, I drop the soymilk.

Day two is the most difficult for me, as the body switches over to ketones. It is most definitely not pleasant, but the intensity does not last. On day three, as I begin autolysis, every semi-recent injury in my body often hurts! Sometimes they hurt a lot (the 'cutting' of the "surgery without the operation"). I've learned that it does not last and that I feel forever better afterwards.

By day three, the blood pressure drops altogether so that one must be vigilant when standing from lying or taking a hot bath. Sit up and adjust. If you get a bit light-headed, it's not a sign you're dying or need to eat. It's normal. Be careful and slowly initiate movements. Rest if you need. Feel. By day four, most discomfort disappears and the pleasure centers of the brain are activated. What an endorphin high!

I don't really notice I'm not eating after that. Really. I hardly think about the fact that I'm not eating. Recently, on a fast of seven days, I had one fresh juice from the local juice bar on the fifth day and approximately every other day, I'd make some fresh, clear, vegetable broth into which I'd dissolve a half-teaspoon of miso and a teaspoon of nutritional yeast. (For electrolytics and B-vitamins.) Otherwise, my main faire is to squeeze a quarter-lemon into a large glass of water or have a pot of herbal tea.

There is a large body of discussion on the matter of enemas, colonics, etc. Play with it. Since my diet is mostly fresh and clean already, I take a tablespoon of psyllium husks on days two and/or three of a fast. This will finish the internal cleansing of the alimentary canal and scrape the last old intestinal hairs/feces out. I may do an enema on days three and/or five as well to finish the cleansing. If I haven't fasted in a while or been an indulgent eater of late, I might treat myself to a colonic as well. (I've had three in the last four decades.) In the end, I think the psyllium husk apporach is best and should always precede (or could be a substitute for) enemas and/or colonics.

Just beware of orthorexics and preachers of this or that. "Only drink _____ water, because....", or "The only true fast is the _____ method,"... etc. "Nature's best diet ..." The body is amazingly flexible and different patterns fit different people and times. When people start talking like that, check the science, evaluate their advice, and grow in your own intelligent, positive choices.

Orthorexia and anorexia are negative in language and action. (Body-negativity is the signature of immature thought...usually followed by sex-negativity and suppression of women.) A fasting program is part of a most positive embrace of life, cooperating with the body in native intelligence, and we mature beyond body-negativity and beyond compelling urgencies.

Aside from psychological issues, we must also ask: Are there people **who should not fast?**

First of all, fasting generally has an adult-only rating. While there are exceptions (particularly with epilepsy), it cannot be recommended for children. Also people with wasting diseases (TB, AIDS, SARS etc) and diabetics should not fast (though some type 2's can benefit under doctor's supervision). Common sense and medical advice tell us that pregnant and nursing mothers should not fast. For a full list of considerations, see the requirements/agreements one must make upon entering a fasting clinic at http://www.fasting.com/whoshouldnotfast.html.

Sometimes between the seventh day and the eleventh, I'll begin to feel an occasional twinge of hunger. Sometimes I eat then, but usually what gets me eating again is that I can't conduct sufficient energy to handle all of life's business.

Someday, I'll take off work when I fast and go for longer. Long-haulers report that the first true hunger begins as early as day 27 but usually comes around day 45! (This is called a 'complete fast.') I am more like Mae West who quipped, "I'm all for restraint, so long as it doesn't go too far."

I know many people talk about how important it is to end your fast "correctly" and I've tried a host of recommendations. If you are trying to change your dietary lifestyle, then there is intelligence to the proposals, but my suggestion is to feel first, think later. I've broken a fast with cheese puffs, though it was something of a joke, but no harm done. My first favorite way was with a baked potato with a dollup of yogurt (a la' Pavlo Arola), but I now usually consume a salad, just less hearty than the one I eat nightly.

What kind of fasting you take up is almost beside the point, only that you intelligently engage a regular dance with hunger. It's similar to what kind of exercise program you do; there may be an optimal one for you, but it is most important that you *engage* it and discover what works for you than to wait until you figure out what's best.

For most of us, learning to fast is like exercise: do an easy version of something you know you can do, then stretch it; slowly intensify it. Or take up a plan, or get an expert to assist you, or _____. The only real question is, will you?

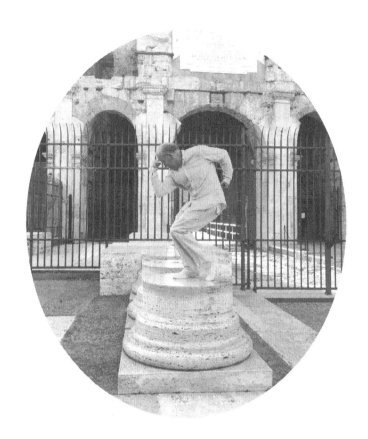

Roman Coliseum, May 2016
(age 64)

## My Grain of Salt

These personal recommendations on adapting to fasting come from forty years of experience and a science teacher's mind. Fortunately, the easy approaches are something that many of us already do from time to time. Now just make it a power.

1. **The eight-hour fast**. A steady "diet" of lengthening the time between two meals showed significant gains in most of the indicators associated with longer fasts. This has always been a proposal of mine, and I found out recently, the hearty recommendation of Bernarr MacFadden as well. Simply stretch the time between meals, *one day a week*, until you get used to it. Many people do this already: when suddenly you realize you haven't eaten all day! Wear it! Grow it! Research on this approach showed maximum gain if the eight hours fell from 11am to 7 pm.

 2. **The 5-2 diet.** Eat like you always do for 5 days, but for 2 days, take in less than 500 calories. That would mean on two days, I would have my morning tea, and only a hearty salad that night. Mosley's books are good and this approach is a great way to start and practice the chosen-hunger-dance. An alternative life-style choice is the Calorie Restriction plan. Daily, eat about 1300 calories. Much cuisine can be shown here as well, but CR without fasting does not deliver some of the

benefits that easier plans give. Google "The CR Way" and "the 5-2 diet" for fuller explanations. [I've over-simplified both plans here. This summary is intended as an introduction. Your own research and preferences are assumed.] Beginning with a "6-1" approach is also a possibile easy beginning.

3. **Paul Bragg's Learning Curve.**  When you have done a couple of full-day fasts (36 hours of juice, broths, teas, and/or just water), make your next goal to do your version of it one day per week for a while. When stability comes with this weekly fast, stretch it once each month to two days, then three. After two or three three-day fasts, the step to a 4-7 day fast is easy. You see, the hardest parts are mostly in the first three days. After that, endorphins kick in and the cleansing exhilarates the body (for the most part). The longer fasts completes the learning  curve and delivers the plural potencies of regeneration and deep cleansing. Paul Bragg recommended three of these longer fasts a year, spring, summer, and autumn. From there, you can make it up as ye see fit.

## Health Practices I Find Most Useful

1. **Live a life devoted to what is unlimited**. This is conducted bodily in harmonious health practices, mentally in study of noble thoughts, and emotionally in passionate living, psychological sensitivities, service in community, and heart-communion. Without this, diet is boring (along with everything else). Because of the severe injuries I have endured, I meditate in an isolation chamber/floatation tank about three times a week for 2-3 hours per session. I can't say enough good things about meditation so I won't. I can say that floating in epsom salts is a great way to take in magnesium, one of the strongest supporters of neural plasticity. I can also praise floating endlessly, for it wonderfully supports my trust and heart-communion with our divine ground and very being.

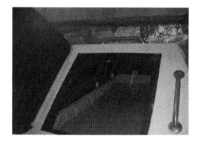

2. **Eat fresher.** This is my singular suggestion for food. There are a thousand 'healthy' diets. I'm sure whatever you're doing is close to one of them. Great. Now take the diet you are already doing and accustomed to and add a bit more freshness — for years... or until you're all raw or discover what's optimum for you. I've done all raw for long periods in my youth, now I'm about 75%, depending on the season.

While I am a flexitarian, meaning I'll eat anything anytime, mostly I am vegan. I think the evolutionary advantages to meat *can* be taken advantage of for the first two decades of life for brain and braun development, but once adulthood is reached, it is best if we then gear flesh-eating down to approximately once a week. Look at your own teeth and digestive system; while it's omni-rific, it's mainly vegetarian. And if you want to reduce your carbon footprint more than home solar and electric vehicles *combined*, it's easy. Eat less meat. For social events, I'll have fish twice a month and I'll eat red meat maybe once every couple of years. I love the Orphic saw: "Don't eat anything that breathes like you do."

3. **Intelligence, not goodness**. I am no advocate for idealistic changes, but have noticed I can slowly (OK too slowly) change to engaging more intelligent ways. This leads me to the lesson I learned from Adi Da about how to be intelligent instead of "good". You see, I am not a "good" person. I'll eat 6 brownies or fresh chocolate cookies before you finish your first one. I'm an unabashed and happy pig. So there is no way I could ever be a good person. I can't not be bad (grammarians smile here). But I *can* add more intelligence. If I eat a larger salad, there is only room for three cookies. "Slowly but slowly," I add fresh enjoyment; I adapt to higher pleasures. For I learned from Adi Da, "Enjoyment is the foundation of the fulfillment of the Law."

4. **Flush**. Drink large amounts of liquid, especially water and teas. I begin my everyday with a super-hydration. (I checked with two urologists.) The hardest part is that I pee like a proverbial sailor for a couple of hours. But I am cleaned out but theses daily flushes. I formulated my tea with the advice of an Aryuvedic pratitioner to be both consoling (my insistence) and healthy. Two bags of Celestial Seasons "Roastaroma", a chickory-root-based mixture, two bags of Green Tea (there is a **large** body of evidence on the health-giving aspects of the polyphenals in green tea, especially their benefits to the endothelial linings of the veins and arteries); a healthy cup of unsweetened soy milk, and stevia (I prefer *Now Foods* "Stevia Glycerite").

   Most days, in order to stimulate the taking in liquids, I'll have a dark piece of the heartiest whole-wheat toast with nothing on it. So beyond my morning tea and toast, I usually don't eat 'til supper and drink moderately. (And I'm quite hungry.) At day's end, I eat a large hearty salad with a cup or brown rice or quinoa, yeast, nuts, seeds, and my own dressing. If my family is having pasta or veggies or pie, I'll have that after my salad. After dinner, I often have my own granola (oats, almond slivers, stevia, soy milk) with berries and soy milk or non-fat yogurt. If my daughter is in a baking cycle, I'm doomed. Ahhh, the advantanges of flexitarianism.

5.  **Exercise**. Like fasting, it's not so important how you do it, the main difference is do you? You can do every other health practice and still not **achieve native radiance** unless you regularly exercise. I try to hike several miles a week, averaging 3 times weekly (twice a week in the winter, 4 times in the summer). At sixty-four, I also still run up stairs instead of elevators; not as a discipline, but as an enjoyment. I am presently recovering from a couple surgeries and have joined a gym for reconstruction. I heartily advocate muscle training and intimacy with machines of all kinds.

6.  **Regular fasting.** <u>Intermittent and Prolonged</u>. Intermittant fasting is something like the 5-2 diet, or my "perpetual Ramadan" (not recommended). Prolonged fasting should slowly work up to the four-day mark to take advantage of pluripotent stem-cell regeneration. It is a fountain of youth.

    I recently had a two and a half hour surgery on my shoulder, fixing three decades of excesses and tears, and was promised a hellish recovery, with strong advice to arrange care for two weeks. Maybe the young surgeon was highly skilled, but after three days, I abandoned the prescribed pain-killers, though I limited my motions to the most gentile and continued to balm my shoulder with regular ice. I was told that less than 5% have such an easy recovery, and usually a youngster who has strong regenerative capacity ...

7. **Hydrotherapy,** or get in the water. Cold water if you can. I know it sounds weird, but subjecting your body to quick bouts of cold is good for you. The research behind this is what is supporting those liquid-nitrogen super-cold container therapies. When you take a cold shower or swim, the shock causes your blood to move from the outer cold to the core of your body, which then bathes your vital organs in fresh blood. Supposedly, this also strengthens your core and immune system. Seems right.
One secret in engaging cold water is to be sensitive to the skin around your eyes. If you splash your face first with cold water, then you won't be as shocked when the rest of your body follows. When finishing a shower, I always turn off the hot and let the cold hit me in the eyes/face and head; then I do the dos-a-dos (and vis-a-vis) for the rest of me. When hiking, I usually splash my face before I jump in streams, lakes, and the ocean — year round. Embrace the stresses! What doesn't kill you, makes you stronger. Wait, that didn't sound quite right.

8. **Stretches**. In addition to exercise, something like yoga gives the body youthfulness. In Aryuveda it is said that you are only as young as your spine (meaning yoga) and your arteries (meaning that the endothelial lining of your veins and arteries should be free of fats and inflammation).

# The Royal Breaths

When you're not feeling well
or happy,
intentionally strengthen some breaths & you will feel better.

\*\*\*\*\*

When you are SCARED,
your breath is frozen,
so take an EVEN & DEEP BREATH.

\*\*\*\*\*

When you are SAD or bored,
your feeling is collapsed, but you can eventually BLOW IT
AWAY.

\*\*\*\*\*

When you are ANGRY or
FRUSTRATED, your feeling is exploding, but you can
BALANCE anger by BREATHING IN really big, (and counting
your blessings).

\*\*\*\*\*

When you are HAPPY, your feeling is free and you can
ENERGIZE your body by BREATHING and RADIATING
HAPPINESS ALL THROUGH YOU.

\*\*\*\*\*

ROYAL STORIES: BREATHING AND FEELING

9. **Breathe deeply**. Breathing is not merely automatic. There are arts and science to respiration as well. The arts of breathing are wonderful and even necessary to learn. A central lesson is how breath and emotions intercourse and interrelate. Not only can we help balance fears, sorrows, and angers by using the breath, we can even breathe in consciously and be inspired.

   On the previous page, you can see my introductory **Royal Breaths** chart for, ahem, children to learn (from *Big Philosophy for Little Kids*, my writing curriculum centered on affective education for elementary-aged children).

10. **Supplements**. I always strive to take in as little as possible. I never take anything all the time. Maybe three-four times a year I'll get rounds of fat-soluble vitamins and build up my reserves (Fish Oils, Vitamins E, D, K2, CoQ10). Since I incorporate nutritional yeast into my rich, everyday diet, I take no multi- or B- vitamins. I often take a minimum amount of aspirin and, in the winter, vitamin C (500 mg, never time-release). But I take no supplement everyday. I take no medicines, save occasional rounds of anti-inflammatories to counter my latest idiocy, I mean, injury.

11. **Oral and skin health.** This is personal and obvious, but worth mentioning. Brush your teeth well and attend to oral health. I gargle and mouth-wash at length every few days as well. In like fashion, I vigorously towel-dry my skin after

bathing, and sun bathe in slanted sunlight. I use oils for my old hands and feet.

12. **Nature**. Being immersed in nature gives great blessings. In nature, we natively and *naturally* intercourse with beauty, which IS our real condition. Reality is beauty itself. This is the truth. Breath this deeply.
    In nature, we more easily feel the substance of life, not its mere mechanics. The mechanics of life are a terrible wheel of pleasure and pain, while the substance of life is divine, which we can feel simply as inherent happiness. This discrimination between the mechanics of life and the substance of life frees feeling and is health-giving.

    Rest in reality. Breathe deeply. Live in beauty.

*"Being led to the things of love is to begin to grow from the beauties of earth and be attracted upwards for the sake of that sacred beauty, that absolute beauty. Our distractions by earthly forms are steps only — so that you go from one beauty to two, seeing beauty in two, and from two to all fair forms, and from fair forms to fair practices and fair notions — until from fair notions one at last arrives at the notion of absolute beauty, and at last knows what beauty is in its very essence. "This, my dear Sokrates," said Diotima, the angel of Mantineia, "is the real life which man should live, in the contemplation of beauty absolute — a beauty which, once beheld, can be seen to utterly surpass the entrancements of gold and embellished garments, or fair boys and young women.*

*"What if one had eyes to see true beauty — divine beauty, I mean; pure and clear and unalloyed, not clogged with the pollutions of mortality and all the colors and vanities of human life. Remember that in communion, beholding beauty with the eye within, one will be enabled to bring forth, not images of beauty, but realities. To see true beauty, one is not beholding an image, but reality."*

— Plato's *Symposium*

Taking on any new skill or manner of being, from the mundane to the spiritual, is well served by "Good Company". Keeping good company is inherently inspirational and instructive. Do not 'believe' in authorities, but rather be inspired by others who have trod the path and sharpen one's discrimination by deeply appreciating the masters of the art.

One of the great voices for fasting and healthy living was Pulitzer Prize winner, Upton Sinclair. This great American author burst onto the American scene in 1906 with his blunt exposure of the conditions in the meat-packing industry with *The Jungle*. He said of this book and its success, "I aimed at the public's heart, and by accident I hit it in the stomach."

An advocate for vegetarianism, even while experimenting with various diets, including steak, Upton Sinclair is famous for his explanation for the disregard of his message: "It is difficult to get a man to understand something, when his salary depends upon his not understanding it."

*The Fasting Cure* (1911) was another bestseller. Sinclair advocated for periodic fasting as being foundational for health. "I had taken several fasts of ten or twelve days' duration, with the result of a complete making over of my health".

What follows is my edit of *The Fasting Cure*. I have not included the lengthy Preface, but the core of the book, 'Perfect Health', is here in entirety. I discarded the section on Death as overwrought, and the rest of the book I edited considerably, with an eye toward the most realistic and discarding testimonials or arguments that needed modern explanation. Still, the provincial and early-scientific voice is to be 'appreciated'.

You can turn the pages of the original book at https://archive.org/details/fastingcure00sinciala.

# The Fasting Cure

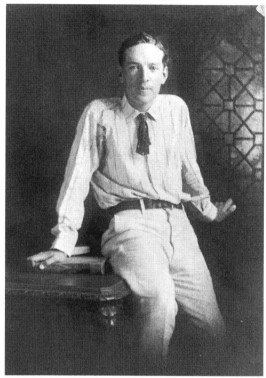

by
**Upton Sinclair**

Dedicated to Bernarr MacFadden
*in cordial appreciation of his personality and teachings*

## *Perfect Health!*

*Have you any conception of what the phrase means? Can you form any image of what would be your feeling if every organ in your body were functioning perfectly? Perhaps you can go back to some day in your youth, when you got up early in the morning and went for a walk, and the spirit of the sunrise got into your blood, and you walked faster, and took deep breaths, and laughed aloud for the sheer happiness of being alive in such a world of beauty. And now you are grown older and what would you give for the secret of that glorious feeling? What would you say if you were told that you could bring it back and keep it, not only for mornings, but for afternoons and evenings, and not as something accidental and mysterious, but as something which you yourself have created, and of which you are completely master?*

*This is not an introduction to a new device in patent medicine advertising. I have nothing to sell, and no process patented. It is simply that for ten years I have been studying the ill health of myself and of the men and women around me. And I have found the cause and the remedy. I have not only found good health, but perfect health; I have found a new state of being, a potentiality of life; a sense of lightness and cleanness and joyfulness, such as I did not know could exist in the human body. "I like to meet you on the street," said a friend the other day. "You walk as if it were such fun!"*

*I look about me in the world, and nearly every body I know is sick. I could name one after another a hundred men and women, who are doing vital work for progress and carrying a cruel handicap of physical suffering. For instance, I am working for social justice, and I have comrades whose help is needed every hour, and they are ill! In one single week's newspapers last spring I read that one was dying of kidney trouble, that another was in hospital from nervous breakdown, and that a third was ill with ptomaine poisoning. And in my correspondence I am told that another of my dearest friends has only a year to live; that another heroic man is a nervous wreck, craving for death; and that a third is tortured by bilious headaches. And there is not one of these people whom I could not cure if I had him alone for a couple of weeks; no one of them who would not in the end be walking down the street "as if it were such fun!"*

*I propose herein to tell the story of my discovery of health, and I shall not waste much time in apologizing for the intimate nature of the narrative. It is no pleasure for me to tell over the tale of my headaches or to discuss my unruly stomach. I cannot take any case but my own, because there is no case about which I can speak with such authority. To be sure, I might write about it in the abstract, and in veiled terms. But in that case the story would lose most of its convincingness, and some of its usefulness. I might tell it without signing my name to it. But there are a great many people who have read my books and will believe what I tell them, who would not take the trouble to read an article without a name. Mr. Horace Fletcher has set us all an example in this matter. He has written several volumes about his individual digestion, with the result that literally millions of people have been helped. In the same way I propose to put my case on record. The reader will find that it is a typical case, for I made about every mistake that a man could make, and tried every remedy, old and new, that anybody had to offer me.*

    *I spent my boyhood in a well-to-do family, in which good eating was regarded as a social grace and the principal interest in life. We had a colored woman to prepare our food, and another to serve it. It was not considered fitting for children to drink liquor, but they had hot bread three times a day, and they were permitted to revel in fried chicken and rich gravies and pastries, fruitcake and candy and ice cream. Every Sunday I would see my grandfather's table with a roast of beef at one end, and a couple of chickens at the other, and a cold ham at one side; at Christmas and Thanksgiving the energies of the whole establishment would be given up to the preparation of delicious foods. And later on, when I came to New York, I considered it necessary to have such food; even when I was a poor student, living on four dollars a week, I spent more than three of it on eatables.*

    *I was an active and fairly healthy boy; at twenty I remember saying that I had not had a day's serious sickness in fourteen years. Then I wrote my first novel, working sixteen or eighteen hours a day for several months, camping out, and living mostly out of a frying pan. At the end I found that I was seriously troubled with dyspepsia* [a combination of indigestion and depression, no longer used since it now makes only a little sense]; *and it was worse the next year, after the second book. I went to see a physician, who gave me some red liquid, which magically relieved the consequences of doing hard brainwork after eating. So I went on for a year or two more, and then I found that the artificially digested food was not being eliminated from my system with sufficient regularity. So I went to another physician, who gave my malady another name and gave me another medicine, and put off the time of reckoning a little while longer.*

*I have never in my life used tea or coffee, alcohol or tobacco; but for seven or eight years I worked under heavy pressure all the time, and ate very irregularly, and ate un-wholesome food. So I began to have headaches once in a while, and to notice that I was abnormally sensitive to colds. I considered these maladies natural to mortals, and I would always attribute them to some specific accident. I would say, "I've been knocking about down town all day"; or, "I was out in the hot sun"; or, "I lay on the damp ground." I found that if I sat in a draught for even a minute I was certain to "catch a cold." I found also that I had sore throat and tonsillitis once or twice every winter; also, now and then, the grippe [flu]. There were times when I did not sleep well; and as all this got worse, I would have to drop all my work and try to rest. The first time I did this a week or two was sufficient but later on a month or two was necessary, and then several months.*

*The year I wrote "The Jungle" I had my first summer cold. It was haying time on a farm, and I thought it was a kind of hay fever. I would sneeze for hours in perfect torment, and this lasted for a month, until I went away to the seashore. This happened again the next summer, and also another very painful experience; a nerve in a tooth died, and I had to wait three days for the pain to "localize," and then had the tooth drilled out, and staggered home, and was ill in bed for a week with chills and fever, and nausea and terrible headaches. I mention all these unpleasant details so that the reader may understand the state of wretchedness to which I had come. At the same time, also, I had a great deal of distressing illness in my family;' my wife seldom had a week without suffering, and my little boy had pneumonia one winter, and croup the next, and whooping-cough in the summer, with the inevitable "colds" scattered in between.*

*After the Helicon Hall fire I realized that I was in a bad way, and for the two years following I gave a good part of my time trying to find out how to preserve my health. I went to Battle Creek, and to Bermuda and to the Adirondacks; I read the books of all the new investigators of the subject of hygiene, and tried out their theories religiously. I had discovered Horace Fletcher a couple of years before. Mr. Fletcher's idea is, in brief, to chew your food, and chew it thoroughly; to extract from each particle of food the maximum of nutriment, and to eat only as much as your system actually needs. This was a very wonderful idea to me, and I fell upon it with the greatest enthusiasm. All the physicians I had known were men who tried to cure me when I fell sick, but here was a man who was studying how to stay well. I have to find fault with Mr. Fletcher's system, and so I must make clear at the outset how much I owe to it. It set me upon the right track--it showed me the goal, even if it did not lead me to it. It made clear to me that all my various ailments were symptoms of one great trouble, the presence in my body of the poisons produced by superfluous and unassimilated food, and that in adjusting the quantity of food to the body's exact needs lay the secret of perfect health.*

*I next read the books of Metchnikoff and Chittenden, who showed me just how my ailments came to be. The unassimilated food lies in the colon, and bacteria swarm in it, and the poisons they produce are absorbed into the system. I had bacteriological examinations made in my own case, and I found that when I was feeling well the number of these toxin-producing germs was about six billions to the ounce of intestinal contents; and when, a few days later, I had a headache, the number was a hundred and twenty billions. Here was my trouble under the microscope, so to speak.*

*These tests were made at the Battle Creek Sanitarium, where I went for a long stay. I tried their system of water cure, which I found a wonderful stimulant to the eliminative organs; but I discovered that, like all other stimulants, it leaves you in the end just where you were. My health was improved at the sanitarium, but a week after I left I was down with the grippe [flu] again.*

*I gave the next year of my life to trying to restore my health. I spent the winter in Bermuda and the summer in the Adirondacks, both of them famous health resorts, and during the entire time I lived an absolutely hygienic life. I did not work hard, and I did not worry, and I did not think about my health except when I had to. I live in the open air all the time, and I gave most of the day to vigorous exercise-- tennis, walking, boating and swimming. I mention this specifically, so that the reader may perceive that I had eliminated all other factors of ill-health, and appreciate to the full my statement that at the end of the year's time my general health was worse than ever before.*

*I was all right so long as I played tennis all day or climbed mountains. The trouble came when I settled down to do brainwork. And from this I saw perfectly clearly that I was over-eating; there was surplus food to be burned up, and when it was not burned up it poisoned me. But how was I to stop when I was hungry? I tried giving up all the things I liked and of which I ate most; but that did no good, because I had such a complacent appetite--I would immediately take to liking the other things! I thought that I had an abnormal appetite, the result of my early training; but how was I ever to get rid of it?*

*I must not give the impression that I was a conspicuously hearty eater. On the contrary, I ate far less than most people eat. But that was no consolation to me. I had wrecked myself by years of overwork, and so I was more sensitive. The other people were going to pieces by slow stages, I could see; but I was already in pieces.*

*So matters stood when I chanced to meet a lady, whose radiant complexion and extraordinary health were a matter of remark to everyone. I was surprised to hear that for ten or fifteen years, and until quite recently, she had been a bed-ridden invalid. She had lived the lonely existence of a pioneer's wife, and had raised a family under conditions of shocking ill health. She had suffered from sciatica and acute rheumatism; from a chronic intestinal trouble which the doctors called "intermittent peritonitis"; chronic catarrh, causing deafness. And this was the woman who rode on horseback with me up Mount Hamilton, in California, a distance of twenty-eight miles, in one of the most terrific rainstorms I have ever witnessed! We had two untamed young horses, and only leather bits to control them with, and we were pounded and flung about for six mortal hours, which I shall never forget if I live to be a hundred. And this woman, when she took the ride, had not eaten a particle of food for four days previously!*

*That was the clue to her escape: she had cured herself by a fast. She had abstained from food for eight days, and all her trouble had fallen from her. Afterwards she had taken her eldest son, a senior at Stanford, and another friend of his, and fasted twelve days with them, and cured them of nervous dyspepsia. And then she had taken a woman friend, the wife of a Stanford professor, and cured her of rheumatism by a week's fast. I had heard of the fasting cure, but this was the first time I had met with it. I was too much burdened with work to try it just then, but I began to read up on the subject--the books of Dr. Dewey, Dr. Hazzard and Mr. Carrington. Coming home from California I got a sunstroke on the Gulf of Mexico, and spent a week in hospital at Key West, and that seemed to give the coup de grave to my long-suffering stomach. After another spell of hard work I found myself unable to digest corn-meal mush and milk; suddenly I was ready for a fast.*

*I began. The fast has become a commonplace to me now; but I will assume that it is as new and as startling to the reader as it was to myself at first, and will describe my sensations at length.*

*I was very hungry for the first day--the un-wholesome, ravening sort of hunger that all dyspeptics* [irritable people with indigestion!] *know. I had a little hunger the second morning, and thereafter, to my very great astonishment, no hunger whatever--no more interest in food than if I had never known the taste of it. Previous to the fast I had had a headache every day for two or three weeks. It lasted through the first day and then disappeared--never to return. I felt very weak the second day, and a little dizzy on arising. I went out of doors and lay in the sun all day, reading; and the same for the third and fourth days--intense physical lassitude, but with great clearness of mind. After the fifth day I felt stronger, and walked a good deal, and I also began some writing. No phase of the experience surprised me more than the activity of my mind: I read and wrote more than I had dared to do for years before.*

*During the first four days I lost fifteen pounds in weight-- something which, I have since learned, was a sign of the extremely poor state of my tissues. Thereafter I lost only two pounds in eight days--an equally unusual phenomenon. I slept well throughout the fast. About the middle of each day I would feel weak, but a massage and a cold shower would refresh me. Towards the end I began to find that in walking about I would grow tired in the legs, and as I did not wish to lie in bed I broke the fast after the twelfth day with some orange juice.*

*I took the juice of a dozen oranges during two days, and then went on the [raw] milk diet, as recommended by Bernarr Macfadden. I took a glassful of warm milk every hour the first day, every three quarters of an hour the next day, and finally every half-hour--or eight quarts a day. This is, of course, much more than can be assimilated, but the balance serves to flush the system out. The tissues are bathed in nutriment, and an extraordinary recuperation is experienced.*

*My sensations on this milk diet were almost as interesting as on the fast. In the first place, there was an extraordinary sense of peace and calm, as if every weary nerve in the body were purring like a cat under a stove. Next there was the keenest activity of mind--I read and wrote incessantly. And, finally, there was a perfectly ravenous desire for physical work. In the old days I had walked long distances and climbed mountains, but always with reluctance and from a sense of compulsion. Now, after the cleaning-out of the fast, I would go into a gymnasium and do work which would literally have broken my back before, and I did it with intense enjoyment, and with amazing results. The muscles fairly leaped out upon my body; I suddenly discovered the possibility of becoming an athlete.*

*I had not taken what is called a "complete" fast--that is, I had not waited until hunger returned. Therefore I began again. I intended only a short fast, but I found that hunger ceased again, and, much to my surprise, I had none of the former weakness. I took a cold bath and a vigorous rub twice a day; I walked four miles every morning, and did light gymnasium work, and with nothing save a slight tendency to chilliness to let me know that I was fasting. I lost nine pounds in eight days, and then went for a week longer on oranges and figs, and made up most of the weight on these.*

*I shall always remember with amusement the anxious caution with which I now began to taste the various foods which before had caused me trouble. Bananas, acid fruits, peanut butter--I tried them one by one, and then in combination, and so realized with a thrill of exultation that every trace of my old trouble was gone. Formerly I had had to lie down for an hour or two after meals; now I could do whatever I chose. Formerly I had been dependent upon all kinds of laxative preparations; now I forgot about them. I no longer had headaches. I went bareheaded in the rain, I sat in cold draughts of air, and was apparently immune to colds. And, above all, I had that marvelous, abounding energy so that whenever I had a spare minute or two I would begin to stand on my head, or to "chin" myself, or do some other "stunt," from sheer exuberance of animal spirits.*

*For several months after this experience I lived upon a diet of raw foods exclusively mainly nuts and fruits. I had been led to regard this as the natural diet for human beings; and I found that so long as I was leading an active life the results were most satisfactory. They were satisfactory also in the case of my wife and still more so in the case of my little boy: the amount of work and bother thus saved in the household may be imagined. But when I came to settle down to a long period of hard and continuous writing, I found that I had not* sufficient bodily energy to digest these raw foods. I resorted to fasting and milk alternately--and that is well enough for a time, but it proves a nervous strain in the end.

### Some Notes on Fasting

*In relation to the article, "Perfect Health," I received some six or eight hundred letters from people who either had fasted, or desired to fast and sought for further information. The letter shared a general uniformity, which made clear to me that I had not been sufficiently explicit upon several important points.*

*The question most commonly asked was how long should one fast, and how one should judge of the time to stop. I personally have never taken a "complete fast," and so I hesitate in recommending this to any one. I have fasted twelve days on two occasions. In both cases I broke my fast because I found myself feeling weak and wanted to be about a good deal. In neither case was I hungry, although hunger quickly returned. I was told by Bernarr Macfadden, and by some of his physicians, that they got their best result from fasts of this length.*

*Of course if a person has started on a fast and it is giving him no trouble, there is no reason why it should not be continued; but I do not in the least believe in a man's setting before himself the goal of a forty or fifty days' fast and making a "stunt" out of it. I do not think of the fast as a thing to be played with in that way. There were several people who wrote me asking about a fast, to whom my reply was that they should simply adopt a rational diet; that I believed their troubles would all disappear without the need of a fast.*

*One should drink all the water he possibly can while fasting, only not taking too much at a time. I take a glass full every hour, at least;*

sometimes every half hour. It is a good plan to drink a great deal of water at the outset, whenever meal time comes around, and one thinks of the other folks beginning to eat.

One should take a bath every day while fasting. I prefer a warm bath followed by a cold shower. Also one should take a small enema. I find a pint of cool water sufficient. I received several letters from people who were greatly disturbed because of constipation during the fast. People apparently do not realize that while fasting there is very little to be eliminated from the body. Of course, there are cases, especially of people who have suffered from long continued intestinal trouble, in which even after three or four weeks the enema continues to bring away quantities of dried and impacted feces.

Many of the questions asked dealt with the manner of breaking the fast. It has been my experience that immediately after a fast the stomach is very weak, and can easily be upset; also the peristaltic muscles are practically without power. It is, therefore, important to choose foods which are readily digested, and also to continue to take the enema daily until the muscles have been sufficiently built up to make a natural movement possible. The thing to do is to take orange juice or grape juice in small quantities for two or three days, and then go gradually upon the milk diet, beginning with half a glass of warm milk at a time. If the milk does not agree with you, you may begin carefully to add baked potatoes and rice and gruels and broths, if you must; but don't forget the enema.

My friend, Mr. Arthur Brisbane, wrote me a gravely disapproving letter when he read that I was fasting. I had a long correspondence with him, at the end of which he acknowledged that there "might be something in it. Even dogs fast when they are ill," he *wrote; and I replied, "I look forward to the time when human beings may be as wise as dogs."*

*The fast is Nature's remedy for all diseases and there are few exceptions to the rule. When you feel sick, fast. Do not wait until the next day, when you will feel stronger, nor till the next week, when you are going away into the country, but stop eating at once. Many of the people who wrote to me were victims of our system of wage slavery, who wrote me that they were ill, but could not get even a few days' release in which to fast. They wanted to know if they could fast and at the same time continue their work. Many can do this, especially if the work is of clerical or routine sort. On my first fast I could not have done any work, because I was too weak. But on my second fast I could have done anything except very severe physical labor. I have one friend who fasted eight days for the first time and who did all her own housework and put up several gallons of preserves on the last day. I have received letters from a couple of women who have fasted ten or twelve days, and have done all their own work. I know of one case of a young girl who fasted thirty-three days and worked at the time at a sanatorium, and on the twenty-fourth day she walked twenty miles.*

### Fasting and the Doctors

*A most discouraging circumstance to me was the attitude of physicians, as revealed in the correspondence that came to me. Mostly I learned of this attitude from the letters of patients who quoted their physicians to me. From the physicians themselves I heard practically nothing. We have some one hundred and forty thousand regularly graduated "medical men" in this country and they are all of them presumably anxious to cure disease. It would seem that an experience such as mine, narrated over my own signature and backed by references to other cases, would have awakened the interest of a good many of these professional men.*

*Out of the six or eight hundred letters that I have received, just two, so far as I can remember, were from physicians; and out of the hundreds of newspaper clippings, which I received, not a single one was from any sort of medical journal. There was one physician, in an out-of-the-way town in Arkansas, who was really interested, and who asked me to let him print several thousand copies of the article in the form of a pamphlet, to be distributed among his patients. One single mind among all the hundred and forty thousand, open to a new truth.*

*Of course I realize what a difficult matter it is for a medical man to face these facts about the fast. Sometimes it seems to me that we have no right to expect their help at all, and that we never will receive it. For we are asking them to destroy themselves, economically speaking.*

*In an article contributed to Physical Culture magazine for January, 1910, I stated that in the course of my search for health I had paid to physicians, surgeons, druggists and sanatoriums not less than fifteen thousand dollars in the last six or eight years. In the last year, since l have learned about the fast, I have paid nothing at all; and the same thing is true, perhaps on a smaller scale, of every one who discovers the fasting cure. As one man who wrote me a letter of enthusiastic gratitude expresses it: "I have spent over five hundred dollars in the last ten years trying to get well on medicines. It cost me only thirty cents to use your method, and for that thirty cents I obtained relief a million-fold more beneficial than from five hundred dollars' worth of medicine."*

### The Humors of Fasting

*At the time of writing these words, it has been just six months since I published my first paper upon fasting, and I am still getting letters about it at the rate of half a dozen a day. The tent which I inhabit is rapidly becoming uninhabitable because of pasteboard boxes full of "fasting-letters" and the storekeeper who is so good as to receive my telegrams over the phone, is growing quite expert at taking down the symptoms of adventurers who get started and want to know how to stop. I could make quite a postage-stamp collection from these letters--I had one from Spain and one from India and one from Argentina all in the same day. I am sure I might have kept a sanatorium for those people who have begged me to let them come and live near me while they were taking a fast.*

*Also, I could fill an article with the "humors" of these letters. One woman writes a long and anxious inquiry as to whether it is permissible to drink any water while fasting; and then follows up with a special delivery letter to say that she hopes I will not think she is crazy--she had read the article again and noted the injunction to drink as much water as she can! And then comes a letter from a man who wants to know if I really mean it all; do I truly expect him to eat nothing whatever--or would I call it fasting if he ate just nuts and fruit now and then? Quite recently I was talking with a physician--a successful and well-known physician--who refused point-blank to believe that a human being could live for more than four or five days without any sort of nutriment. There was no use talking about it--it was a physiological impossibility; and even when I offered him the names and addresses of a hundred people who had done it, he went off unconvinced. And yet that same physician professes a religion which through nearly two thousand years has recommended "fasting and prayer" as the method of the soul's achievement; and he will go to church and listen reverently to accounts of a forty-day fast in the wilderness! And he lives in a country in which there are sanatoriums where hundreds of people are fasting all the time, and where twenty or thirty-day fasts occasion no more remark than a good golf score at a summer hotel!*

*When I was a very small boy, I recall that Dr. Tanner took a forty-day fast in a museum in New York; and I recollect well the conversation in our family--how obvious it was that the thing must be a fake, and how foolish people were to be taken in by so absurd a fake. "He gets something to eat when nobody's looking," we would say.*

*But then what about his weight? Here is a man, going along day by day, year in and year out, weighing in the neighborhood of a hundred and fifty pounds; and now, all of a sudden, he begins to lose a pound a day, as regularly as the sun rises. How does he do it? "Well," we would say, "he must work hard and get rid of it."*

*But how can a man do that, when he had no longer enough muscular tissue left to support his weight? and when his pulse is only thirty-five beats to the minute?*

*It must be a curious experience to go for three months without tasting food. It is no wonder that the stomach and all the organs of assimilation forget how to do their work. The one danger in the fasting treatment is that when you break the fast, hunger is apt to come back with a rush, while, on the other hand, the stomach is weak, and the utmost caution is needed. If you yield to your cravings, you may fill your whole system with toxins, and undo all the good of the treatment; but if you go slowly, and restrict yourself to very small quantities of the most easily assimilated foods, then in an incredibly short time the body will have regained its strength.*

*I was interested enough in the question of fasting to spend some time at a sanatorium where they make a specialty of it. One can see a sicker looking collection of humans in such a place than anywhere else in the world, I fancy. In the first place, people do not take the fasting cure until they are looking desperate; and when they have got into the fast they look more desperate. At the later stages they sometimes take to wheelchairs; and at all times they move with deliberation, and their faces wear serious expressions. They gather in little groups and discuss their symptoms; there is nothing so interesting in the world when you are fasting as to talk symptoms with a lot of people who are doing the same thing. There are some who are several days ahead of you, and who make you ashamed of your doubts and others who are behind you, and to whom you have to appear as an old campaigner. So you develop an esprit de corps, as it were, though that sounds as if I were trying to make a pun.*

*All this may not seem very alluring; but it is far better than a lifetime of illness, such as many of these people have known before. I never knew that there was such terrible suffering in the world until I heard some of their stories; they would indeed be depressing company, were it not for the fact that now they are getting well. The reader may answer sarcastically that they think they are. I have talked with not less than a hundred people who have fasted for three days or more, and out of these there were but two or three who did not report themselves as greatly benefited. So I am accustomed to say that I would rather spend my time in a fasting sanatorium than in an ordinary "swell" hotel. The people in the former are making themselves well and know it; while the people in the latter are making themselves ill, and don't know it.*

### A Symposium on Fasting

*Recently I published a request that those who had tried the fast as the result of my advocacy would write to advise me of the results. I stated that I desired to hear unfavorable results as well as favorable; that I wanted to get at the facts, and would tabulate the results exactly as they came. The questions asked were as follows:*

*1. How many times have you fasted?* □

*2. How many days on each occasion?*

*3. From what complaints did you suffer?*

*4. Were these complaints ever diagnosed by regular physician? If so, give the names and addresses of these physicians.*

*5. Do you consider that you were definitely benefited by the fasts? If so, in what way?*

*6. For how long did the benefit continue?*

*7. Do you consider that you were completely cured?*

*8. Do you consider that you were definitely harmed? If so, in what way?*

*9. Have you ever been examined by any regular physician since the cure? If so, give name and address.*

*10. Are you willing that your name and address should be quoted for the benefit of others?*

*The total number of fasts taken was 277, and the average number of days was 6. There were 90 of five days or over, 51 of ten days or over, and 6 of 30 days or over. Out of the 109 persons who wrote to me, 100 reported benefit, and 17 no benefit. Of these 17, about half give wrong breaking of the fast as the reason for the failure. In cases where the cure had not proved permanent, about half mentioned that the recurrence of the trouble was caused by wrong eating, and about half of the rest made this quite evident by what they said. Also it is to be noted that in the cases of the 17 who got no benefit, nearly all were fasts of only three or four days.*

*Dora Jordan, Connersville, Md. Indigestion, extreme nervousness, neuralgia in its worst form. Fasted thirty days, did most of cooking for a family of five, was at no time tempted to eat. "I am no longer troubled with the old diseases, and weigh more than ever before. After my fast I felt as happy and care free as a little child."*

*C.L. Clark, Greenville, Mich. Nervous, poor digestion. Fasted nine days. "I have been wonderfully benefited, and am a rabid convert. Alas, for the poor mortal who shows the faintest spark of interest in my fast--I hand him the whole works, lock, stock and barrel! I feel a new power and new incentive in life. Whenever I see a sick person, I feel like telling him that for all he knows to the contrary, good health has been and may be only eight or ten days away and waiting for years for him to claim it."*

*Gordon G. Ives, 147 Forsythe Bldg., Fresno, Cal. "Have fasted a good many times since 1899, to cure catarrh of stomach, constipation, deafness of four months' standing, neuralgia, etc. Duration: from one to sixteen days. Never failed in accomplishing a cure. Benefit continued until I had over-eaten for a long time. Complaints were never diagnosed by regular physicians, as I got on to them in 1894. Use my name if it will help the truth."*

*Mrs. Maria L. Scott, Boring, Ariz. Reports case of husband, who fasted seven days for constipation and deafness; had been obliged to take enema daily for several months. Complete cure.*

*Mrs. Mae Bramble, Alba, Pa., R. F. D. 70. One fast of thirty days, another of three days; nervous prostration the first time, appendicitis the second time. "The first complaint was diagnosed, the second was not; as I am a professional nurse, I understood the symptoms myself." Complete and permanent cure. "I have never had a return of the nervous trouble, and am well of the other complaint. It is five years since the first fast."*

*E.B. Bayne, White Plains, N.Y. Sends record of fasts taken by two people, Mr. and Mrs. A. Mr. A. fasted for rheumatism, which had caused kidney and bladder trouble of years' standing, and iritis; fasted five days and the four days and was completely cured. Mrs. A. Neuralgia and catarrhal deafness. Completely cured. "Finds that exposure to draughts has no effect upon her whatever, heretofore she would catch cold upon the least exposure."*

*Mrs. Charles H. Vosseller, Newark, N. J. "I don't agree with you or Bernarr Macfadden in not recommending fasting for tuberculosis. My case was diagnosed by Dr. B. G--, New Brunswick, N.J. I fasted nineteen days and was completely cured; I received no harm, and have been examined since by a physician. I weigh 114 lbs. now and before my fast weighted 100 lbs. I never felt better in my life than I do at present. Do not know that I have a pair of lungs."*

### Fasting and the Mind

*The reader will observe that I discuss this fasting question from a materialistic viewpoint. I am telling what it does to the body; but besides this, of course, fasting is a religious exercise. I heard the other day from a man who was taking a forty-day fast, as a means of increasing his "spiritual power." I am not saying that for you to smile at--he has excellent authority for the procedure. The point with me is that I find life so full of interest just now that I don't have much time to think about my "soul." I get so much pleasure out of a handful of raisins, or a cold bath, or a game of tennis, that I fear it is interfering with my spiritual development.*

*I have, however, a very dear friend who goes in for the things of the soul, and she tells me that when you are fasting, the higher faculties are in a sensitive condition, and that you can do many interesting things with your subliminal self. For instance, she had always considered herself a glutton; and so, during an eight-day fast, just before doing to sleep and just after awakening, she would lie in a sort of trance and impress upon her mind the idea of restraint in eating. The result, she declared, has been that she has never since then had an impulse to over-eat.*

*There are many such curious things, about which you may read in the books of the yogis and the theosophists--who were fasting in previous incarnations when you and I were swinging about in the treetops by our tails.*

*The great thing about the fast is that it sets you a new standard of health. You have been accustomed to worrying along somehow; but now you discover your own possibilities, and thereafter you are not content until you have found some way to keep that virginal state of stomach which one possesses for a month or two after a successful fast. It must mean, of course, many changes in your life, if you really wish to keep it. It means the giving up of tobacco and alcohol, and a too sedentary life, and steam-heated rooms; above all else, it means giving up self-indulgent eating.*

---

## Also by Frank Marrero

*Lincoln Beachey: The Man Who Owned the Sky*

*Recollections of Sokrates*

*Big Philosophy for Little Kids: Writing with Character*

*Deep Roots: Illuminations in Etymology*

*The View from Delphi: Rhapsodies of Hellenic Wisdom and an Ecstatic Appreciation of Western History*

*A Monkey's Tale for the Divine Person: Leelas in Praise of Avatar Adi Da Samraj*

forthcoming

*Telling Fish About Water: On the Process of Perception and Seeing the Truth*

*The Early Life Adventures of Frankie Free Boy: Naive Tales from a Most Ridiculous Life*

www.frankmarrero.com

## About the Author

Frank Marrero lives just north of San Francisco's Golden Gate and teaches elementary children in inner city schools. He is the proud father of Ella (17) and Salem (21), and loves to fast, hike, and write.

In his native Tennessee, Frank first encountered Adi Da in 1976 and two years later, just after his 26th birthday, Frank sold his businesses and home to live near Adi Da's ashram. Adi Da brought Frank into his intimate sphere, blessing Frank with fiery illuminations and nectarous sublimities.

Adi Da's freedom relieved Frank of all orthorexcia, all shoulds and shouldn'ts, so that consideration and feeling, not mere ideas and thinking, could more easily be one's guide.

Adi Da also charged Frank to study the pre-Socratic mystery traditions for a decade and write about it. This passion continues as his life's work.

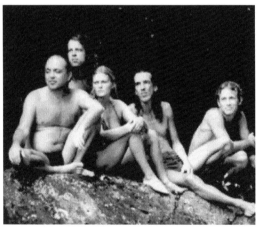

*Adi Da far left, author far right, 1982*